Eucharistic Ministry to the Sick

Marie Zoglman, ASC

**Santa Clara University
Pastoral Ministries Program
Sheed & Ward
Kansas City**

Copyright© 1996 by Marie Zoglman

All rights reserved. No part of this book may be reproduced or transmitted in any form or by any means, electronic or mechanical, including photocopying, recording or by an information storage and retrieval system without permission in writing from the Publisher.

Sheed & Ward™ is a service of The National Catholic Reporter Publishing Company.

ISBN 1-55612-952-1

Published by: Sheed & Ward
115 E. Armour Blvd.
P.O. Box 419492
Kansas City, MO 64141-6492

To order, call: (800) 333-7373

Contents

Introduction 1

One
A Restored Tradition 5
   The Early Church Tradition 5
   The Movement Away From the Early Church Tradition . . 8
   The Restoration of the Early Church Tradition 11

Two
Analysis of *The Rite of Communion of the Sick* 17
   The Symbolic Actions of Rite of *Communion of the Sick* . 19
   The Prayer Texts of the Rite of *Communion of the Sick* . . 27
   The Lectionary of the Rite of *Communion of the Sick* . . . 32

Three
A Catechetical Process for Preparing Ministers to the Sick . 35
   Introduction 35
   Session One: The Community Reaches Out in Compassion 37
   Session Two: The Community Listens and Responds in Faith . 52
   Session Three: The Community Unites in Celebrative Sharing 66
   Session Four: The Community Reflects and Prays Together 77

Conclusion 84
   The History of the Rite 84
   Theological Reflection on the Rite 84
   The Structural Study of the Rite 85
   The Catechetical Method 85

Appendix A: Analysis of Prayer Texts and Dialogical Exchanges 87

Appendix B: Lectionary Analysis 91

Appendix C: Human Sickness and Its Meaning in the Mystery of Salvation 93

Appendix D: Outline of the Rite 95

Appendix E: Visual Aid for Session Two 96

Appendix F: Discussion Questions 97

Appendix G: A Brief List of Resources for Those Who Visit Persons with HIV or AIDS 98

Bibliography 100

Acknowledgments

I am grateful to my religious congregation, Adorers of the Blood of Christ, for its continuing support. I am also indebted to the faculty of the Graduate Program in Pastoral Ministries at Santa Clara University especially Rita Claire Dorner, O.P. and Anne Marie Mongoven, O.P.

Introduction

In response to the Last Supper command of Jesus, "Do this as a remembrance of me" (Lk. 22:19), the community of believers celebrates the Eucharist. The faithful gather "to listen to the Word and to pray so that, remembering and giving thanks, [they] may share the Lord's Supper and so be ready to know and to do the Lord's work."[1] Through the power of the Holy Spirit, Christ is present in these actions of the assembly.[2] In receiving the holy gifts of the eucharistic celebration, the People of God are united to Christ and to one another.

From its table of celebration, the church sends members of the assembly to the sick. This practice of the church, taking communion to the sick, is a powerful symbol of the unity between the local faith community and its sick members. "In receiving the body and blood of Christ, the sick are united sacramentally to the Lord and are reunited with the Eucharistic community from which illness has separated them."[3]

Because "the faithful who are ill are deprived of their rightful and accustomed place in the Eucharistic community,"[4] the church commis-

---

1. James Dallen, *Gathering for Eucharist: A Theology of Sunday Assembly* (Daytona Beach: Pastoral Arts Associate of North America, 1982), 59-60.

2. Vatican II, "The Constitution on the Sacred Liturgy," in *Vatican Council II: The Conciliar and Post Conciliar Documents*, Vol. 1, ed. Austin Flannery, O. P. (Northport: Costello Publishing Company, 1990), 7. (Hereafter referred to as CSL with paragraph number.)

3. Congregation for Divine Worship, "Pastoral Care of the Sick: Rites of Anointing and Viaticum," Part I, in *The Rites of the Catholic Church*, International Commission on English in the Liturgy (New York: The Pueblo Publishing Company, 1990), Intro. 51. (Hereafter referred to as PCS with paragraph number.)

4. Congregation for Divine Worship, "The Rite of Communion of the Sick in Ordinary Circumstances," in *The Rites of the Catholic Church*, International Commission on English in the Liturgy (New York: The Pueblo Publishing Company, 1990), 73. (Hereafter referred to as RCS with paragraph number.)

sions special Eucharistic ministers to care for the sick. These Eucharistic ministers are sent to take the word and Eucharist to the sick members of the assembly. *The Rite of Communion to the Sick in Ordinary Circumstances* (RCS) explains:

> In bringing communion to them the ministers of communion represent Christ and manifest faith and charity on behalf of the whole community toward those who cannot be present at the Eucharist. For the sick the reception of communion is not only a privilege but also a sign of support and concern shown by the Christian community for its members who are ill (RCS 73).

This specific pastoral and sacramental care of the sick is the obligation of the Eucharistic assembly. The RCS states:

> Priests with pastoral responsibilities should see to it that the sick or aged, even though not seriously ill or in danger of death, are given every opportunity to receive the Eucharist frequently, even daily, especially during the Easter season. . . To provide frequent communion for the sick, it may be necessary to ensure that the community has sufficient number of ministers of communion (RCS 72).

The provision of sufficient ministers implies preparation of these ministers for the task of this ministry. This resource meets this need by offering a liturgical catechetical process to prepare Eucharistic ministers for the pastoral care of the sick.

Alongside the general training that is provided, some attention is given to the unique needs of those living with HIV and AIDS, as this disease presents particular pastoral challenges and opportunities that all well-trained eucharistic ministers should be made aware of. As the Bishops of the California Catholic Conference wrote in their 1987 pastoral letter on AIDS, "A Call to Compassion":

> There were no conditions placed on Jesus' expression of concern for the outcasts and the wounded of His world. If we are to follow His example, our response to those who are ill should be that of compassion, not of judgment. . . . We are called to respond with that same love for those who in our day suffer from this new and deadly disease of AIDS. . . . By providing direct care, by visiting, by offering our prayers, and by sharing in the Eucharist and the Sacrament of Anointing, we can offer our companionship, along with the refreshment and reconciliation of the Lord.

Ministry to the sick is one of the oldest ministries of the church. It began with Jesus. He "went about doing good and healing all" (Acts 10:38). The church continues this mission of Jesus. Throughout its history, the church has shown concern for the sick. In recent years, the church formulated this solicitude in its revised ritual: *The Pastoral Care of the Sick: Rites of Anointing and Viaticum.*

In Chapter Two, *The Rite of Communion of the Sick in Ordinary Circumstances* (RCS 71-91) is set forth. This rite is the basis for a catechesis to prepare Eucharistic ministers to take communion to the sick found in this resource.

In Chapter One, we will explore the three historical phases of the practice of the laity participating in Eucharist and taking communion to the sick. The first phase is the early church tradition which included taking communion to the sick. The gradual movement away from the participation of the laity in Eucharist and, thus, from being allowed to take communion to the sick constitutes the second phase. The third phase is the restoration of the early tradition of the church encouraging participation of the assembly in Eucharist and sending members of the assembly to the sick.

Chapter Two contains the analysis of *The Rite of Communion of the Sick in Ordinary Circumstances.* The analysis of this rite focuses on its ritual components: the symbolic action, the prayer texts, and specific lectionary texts. The analysis of each ritual component includes: a description of the component, the method of analysis, the summation of the analysis, and a conclusion which addresses how the analysis helps shape the preparation of Eucharistic ministers to the sick.

Chapter Three sets out the creative design of liturgical catechesis for Eucharistic ministers preparing to take communion to the sick. Each of the four catechetical sessions is based on a specific part of *The Rite of Communion of the Sick in Ordinary Circumstances.* Session One, "The Community Reaches Out in Compassion," centers on the Introductory Rites of gathering. Session Two, "The Community Listens and Responds in Faith," focuses on the Liturgy of the Word. Session Three, "The Community Unites in Celebrative Sharing," focuses on the Liturgy of Holy Communion. The final Session, "The Community Reflects and Prays Together," considers how ministry to the sick affects the faith life of the ministers.

The catechetical sessions designed to prepare ministers to the sick form the core of this paper. They owe their inspiration to the catechetical process taught by Rita Claire Dorner, O.P. in Pastoral Liturgy and Anne

Marie Mongoven, O.P. in Catechetics at the Graduate Program in Pastoral Ministry at Santa Clara University. Guided by their vision, the sessions reflect the substance and spirit of their teaching.

This presentation is based upon the following primary sources: *The Rite of Communion of the Sick in Ordinary Circumstances* (RCS 71-91); "The Constitution on the Sacred Liturgy" (CSL); *The Lectionary of the Rite*; and, *And You Visited Me: Sacramental Ministry to the Sick and Dying* by Charles W. Gusmer.[5]

---

5. Charles W. Gusmer, *And You Visited Me: Sacramental Ministry to the Sick and Dying, Studies in the Reformed Rites of the Catholic Church*, Vol. 4 (New York: Pueblo Publishing Company, 1989).

ONE

A Restored Tradition

As background for the catechesis of Eucharistic ministers to the sick, it would serve well to first address the existence of this ministry in the church. Modern-day Catholics think of special ministers of communion as a new ministry. Actually, the recent new practice of Eucharistic ministers to the sick is an old tradition restored to meet the pastoral needs of our day. The history of the eucharistic practices rooted in the early church tradition reveals two parallel trends: the participation of the assembly in Eucharist and taking communion to the sick from the Eucharistic assembly.

This chapter considers three historical phases of these parallel trends which have direct bearing on the ministry to the sick. In the early church phase, the laity participated in the Eucharist, which included taking communion to the sick. The second historical phase saw a gradual movement away from lay participation in the Eucharist and, thus, in the laity taking communion to the sick.

In the recent restoration of the early church tradition, the church encourages participation of the assembly in Eucharist and sends representatives to take communion to sick members.

The Early Church Tradition

The early Judeo Christians "went to the temple area together every day, while in their homes they broke bread" (Acts 2:46). As their usual practice, they continued to attend the Sabbath service at the synagogue. This consisted of scripture reading, and the singing of psalms in praise of God. In their home gatherings, the early church community celebrated Eucharist; that is, as part of a meal, they broke bread in the name of Jesus. It was "with exultant hearts they ate these meals, praising God and enjoying favor with all the people" (Acts 2:46-47).

According to Joseph Jungmann's study, *The Mass of the Roman Rite: Its Origins and Development*,[1] the *First Apology* of Justin is the first full account of a Christian Eucharist.[2] Justin's account of the Sunday celebration states:

> ... We offer prayers in common for ourselves, for the newly baptized, and for all others all over the world .... When we finish praying, we greet one another with a kiss. Then bread and a cup of wine mixed with water are brought to him who presides over the brethren. He takes them and offers prayers glorifying the Father of the universe through the name of the Son and of the Holy Spirit, and he utters a lengthy thanksgiving because the Father has judged us worthy of these gifts. When the prayers and Eucharist are finished, all the people present give their assent with an "Amen!" "Amen!" in Hebrew meaning "So be it!" When the president has finished his Eucharist and the people have all signified their assent, those whom we call "deacons" distribute the bread and the wine and water over which the Eucharist has been spoken, to each of those present; they also carry them to those who are absent.[3]

In his commentary on Justin, Jungmann notes the emphasis on the congregation's Amen, which strongly confirms the thanksgiving spoken by the presider. For Jungmann, the community spirit of oneness is expressed in a celebration with the character of a meal. The reception of communion unites the entire community, even those who are absent.[4]

Nathan Mitchell points out that Justin's *First Apology* is the first literary account of the custom of carrying communion to those absent from the Eucharistic assembly. He writes:

> ... it witnesses to a custom of long duration in the church: the taking of communion to those unable to attend the Eucharistic assembly .... Justin's report is significant because it provides the earliest evidence for a distribution of the Eucharist outside the immediate celebration of the liturgy itself. At the same time, however, the intimate connection between Sunday worship and communion outside of Mass is evident: the deacons appear to

---

1. Joseph A. Jungmann, S.J., *The Mass of the Roman Rite: Its Origins and Development*, Vol. I, trans. Francis A. Brunner, C.S.S.R. (Westminster: Christian Classics, Inc., 1986), 20.
2. Ibid., 22.
3. Justin Martyr, "First Apology," in *Springtime of the Liturgy*, Lucien Deiss, C.S.Sp. (Collegeville: The Liturgical Press, 1979), 65.
4. Jungmann, 23.

proceed directly from the assembly to to the distribution of gifts to those absent.[5]

In the early church, the day for the community celebration of the Eucharist was Sunday.[6] Paul celebrated with the congregation at Troas "on the first day of the week . . . . he broke bread and ate" (Acts 20:7-11). The text of the oldest Eucharistic prayer in the Christian tradition, the *Didache,* explains: "From the very beginning, Sunday, which is the memorial day of the resurrection, has been linked to the celebration of the Eucharist."[7] Justin Martyr concurs in his *First Apology:* "On the day named after the sun, all who live in city or countryside assemble."[8] Finally, at the beginning of the fourth century, this practice of celebrating Eucharist on Sunday was "formulated as a sanctioned command at the Council of Elvira."[9]

Since the celebration of Mass occurred on Sunday, it was customary for the faithful to take sufficient supply of consecrated bread home. The *Apostolic Tradition* of Hippolytus (ca. 215) clearly witnesses to this private reservation of the Eucharist in the homes of Christians.[10] Hippolytus gives instruction to receive the Eucharist before eating food and to reverence the Eucharist:

> Each believer is to take care to receive the Eucharist before tasting anything else. For if he receives it with faith, and then some deadly poison is given to him afterwards, it will not have power to harm him (36).

> Each person must see to it that an unbeliever, or a mouse or other animal, does not eat the Eucharist, and no part of it falls to the ground and is lost. For it is the body of the Lord that the faithful eat, and they must not treat it with contempt (37).[11]

This domestic form of reservation and reception of Eucharist involved neither ordained ministers nor official rites.[12] This practice made

---

5. Nathan Mitchell, O.S.B., *Cult and Controversy: The Worship of the Eucharist Outside Mass* (New York: Pueblo Publishing Company, 1982), 10-11.

6. Jungmann, 245.

7. "Didache," in *Springtime of the Liturgy,* Lucien Deiss, C.S.Sp. (Collegeville: The Liturgical Press, 1979), 14.

8. Justin Martyr, *First Apology,* 67.

9. Jungmann, 245.

10. Mitchell, 11.

11. Hippolytus of Rome, *The Apostolic Tradition,* in *Springtime of the Liturgy,* Lucien Deiss, C.S.Sp. (Collegeville: The Liturgical Press, 1979), 36-37.

12. Mitchell, 15.

it possible for the sick, prisoners, and isolated monks to communicate frequently, even daily.[13]

History also evidences the reception of Eucharist in the hand. Champlin cites several examples of proof for this assertion. Speaking to a group of newly baptized Christians in 348, St. Cyril, the bishop of Jerusalem, outlined the proper way to receive Communion: ". . . make your left hand a throne for the right one, which is to receive the King. . . ."[14] St. Theodore of Mopsuestia commented: "Everyone stretches out his (sic) right hand to receive the Eucharist which is given and puts his left hand under it."[15] Around 570, St. John of Damascus observed: "Making the figure of the cross with our hands, we receive the body of Christ crucified."[16] Finally, a sacramentary of the ninth century contained a Communion scene showing Eucharist placed in the communicant's hands.[17] The customs, then, of the laity touching, holding, and distributing the consecrated bread, and drinking from the cup, have deep roots in the Catholic tradition. Although the practice of taking Eucharist home for daily reception, for the sick, and for protection from evil declined after the fourth century, this custom continued until the seventh or eighth century.[18]

The Movement Away from the Early Church Tradition

Why did these customary practices for receiving communion begin changing in the early Middle Ages? According to Mitchell, the underlying cause was a changing attitude about the Eucharist and liturgical worship:

> . . . a decisive shift in liturgical sensibility appears in the fourth century. . . . Important changes in both ritual action and ritual interpretation become noticeable. Gestures of reverence and adoration emerge at the point in the Mass when people are invited to communion . . . . Increasingly the Eucharist is interpreted as ritual drama . . . the solemn rehearsal of Jesus' life, death and resurrection . . . . The altar is regarded not so much a table but

---

13. Joseph M. Champlin, *An Important Office of Immense Love: A Handbook for Eucharistic Ministers* (New York: Paulist Press, 1984), 7.
14. Ibid.
15. Ibid., 8.
16. Ibid.
17. Ibid.
18. Mitchell, 18.

as a tomb where Jesus is laid and then resurrected through liturgical action. . . . Ceremonial gestures of reverence toward the reserved Eucharist appear as it is used within . . . liturgy. In short, the communal symbols of gathering at table to eat and drink with thanksgiving have become ritual dramas of watching Jesus' tomb while the priest pronounces sacred words that confect a sacrament.[19]

Concurring with Mitchell, Joseph Champlin points to the emphasis on the divine aspects of the Eucharist: "The real, holy, awesome presence of Christ our God in the sacrament" was stressed. "The host was, in a way, to be adored more than to be eaten."[20] William Belford characterizes this mindset in the church: "Respect for the sacrament replaced hunger for it, adoration and awe took the place of participation and communion."[21]

This distorted attitude toward Eucharist and liturgical worship affected the frequency of reception of communion by the laity. Until the fourth century, the faithful generally received communion at every Mass. For believers, receiving the Lord's body and blood formed an integral and natural part of every celebration of eucharist. But as the divinity of Christ began to dominate Christian thinking, the people lost hold of this traditional practice. A heightened sense of personal unworthiness of this sublime gift led to infrequent reception of communion.

Different penitential disciplines and the prevailing attitude toward Eucharist were other influences that discouraged frequent communion. In the tenth century, sacramental confession became an obligation before each reception of Eucharist. Preparation required longer and stricter fast. The observance of continence became an additional requirement for married people. The notion that frequent gazing upon the Eucharist could in some way replace the sacramental reception prevailed after the end of the twelfth century. A justification for the practice of infrequent communion in the Middle Ages was that the priest received communion as representative of the entire community.[22]

The manner of reception of Eucharist also affected the shift in attitude toward the Eucharist. The ordinary custom of receiving

---

19. Ibid., 61-62.
20. Champlin, 9.
21. William J. Belford, *Special Ministers of the Eucharist* (Collegeville: The Liturgical Press, 1990), 10.
22. Joseph A. Jungmann, S.J., *The Mass of the Roman Rite: Its Origins and Development*, Vol. II, trans. Francis A. Brunner, C.S.S.R. (Westminster: Christian Classics, Inc., 1986), 360-364.

communion in the hand changed to the practice of placing the sacred host on the tongue. The concern over possible misuse and, more strongly, the growing respect for the Eucharist, led to this change. This new method of receiving was decreed by the Council of Rouen (ca. 878): "Let not the Eucharist be put in the hand of any lay man or woman, but only in the mouth." This change of custom occurred at the same time as the transition from leavened to unleavened bread. Jungmann suggests that the thin wafer would more easily adhere to the moist tongue.[23]

The custom of receiving from the chalice survived longer than communion in the hand. In the West, the fear of spilling the Precious Blood led to a change from drinking directly from the chalice to receiving through a silver or golden tube. Some preferred intinction, the dipping of the Bread into the Wine. However, intinction was not approved in the West. This disapproval played a role in a more radical development. Withholding the chalice from the faithful became the practice during the thirteenth century. Thomas Aquinas (d.1274) described this new change as the well-founded custom of some churches.[24]

These changes gradually excluded the laity from taking communion to the sick. Such prohibitions began in the seventh century and grew more numerous in the ninth century. Local councils and synods objected to lay persons acting as ministers of communion. For example, the Council in Trullo (692) forbade the laity to distribute communion whenever a bishop, presbyter, or deacon was present. In the West, the Council of Rouen implicitly prohibited Eucharistic reservation by the laity in their homes and taking communion to the sick.[25]

Even in the Middle Ages, however, councils and synods recognized that in cases of extreme necessity the laity could function as ministers of communion for the sick and dying. The Council of Westminster (1138) exemplifies this: "We decree that the body of Christ be taken to the ill only by a priest or deacon; but in case of pressing necessity it may be taken, with great reverence, by anyone."[26] Yet, the legislation of the Latin church did not include the laity as possible ministers of communion in cases of necessity. The 1917 Code of Canon Law (canon 845) states:

---

23. Ibid., 381-382.
24. Thomas Aquinas, as quoted in Jungmann, 382-385.
25. Mitchell, 276-278.
26. W.H. Freestone, *The Sacrament Reserved* "Alcuin Club Collections, XXI," (London: A.R. Mowbray and Co.,1917), 56-57, quoted in *Cult and Controversy: The Worship of the Eucharist Outside of Mass*, Nathan Mitchell, 279-280.

The ordinary minister of holy communion is the priest alone; the extraordinary [minister] is the deacon, if permission has been granted, for a grave reason, by the local ordinary or the pastor; in case of necessity [the permission] may legitimately be presumed.[27]

The increasing restrictions on ministry to the sick and the less frequent reception of communion were signs of a progressive decline in active participation of the faithful in the celebration of Eucharist in the Middle Ages. In *The Eucharist*, Robert Cabie notes other factors that contributed to the increased distance between the priest at the altar and the assembly. Cabie points to the abandonment of the donation of the gifts of the faithful, the multiplication of private Masses, and the use of Latin, which was inaccessible to the ordinary lay worshipers during this time.[28]

The monastic character the liturgy had acquired added to the lack of involvement of the congregation. Because the chanting became complex, the "choir" replaced the congregation. Actual physical barriers such as the installation of screens further indicated a separation between the faithful and the few responsible for the celebration of Eucharist. The laity became onlookers so passive that the liturgical books no longer mention their presence.[29]

The Restoration of the Early Church Tradition

The liturgical reform of the nineteenth century sought to bring change in the worship life of the people. The monks at Solesmes, Beuron, Maria Laach, and Louvain attempted to discover and recover some of the liturgical practices of the past.[30] For example, Lambert Beauduin approached renewal through practical and pastoral endeavors: the translation of the Roman missal for the use of the faithful, a liturgical orientation of all Catholic piety to be based on the Mass and the prayer of the divine office, the promotion of Gregorian chant, and efforts to edu-

---

27. As quoted in *Cult and Controversy: The Worship of the Eucharist Outside Mass*, Nathan Mitchell, 281.
28. Robert Cabie, *The Eucharist*, trans. Matthew J. O'Connell, *The Church at Prayer*, Vol. II, ed. A.G. Martimort (Collegeville: The Liturgical Press, 1986), 139.
29. Ibid.
30. Champlin, 11.

cate priests to engender support for renewal at the parish level.[31] Such grassroots efforts provided a theological basis and practical impetus for restoring the laity's part in liturgy.

Pius X gave papal approval and support. His decree on sacred music, *The Restoration of Church Music* (November 22, 1903), called for reforms and urged the involvement of lay persons in the sacred liturgy. He declared that the "most important and indispensable source" of "the true Christian spirit" is the faithful's "active participation in the most sacred mysteries and in the public and solemn prayer of the Church."[32] This officially ushered in the trend of restoring the laity to their rightful place in worship.

In a continued effort to restore a proper celebration of Eucharist, Pius X published the encyclical *Quam Singulari*, (December 22, 1905). To change the past pattern of infrequent communion, Catholics were specifically encouraged to approach the table of Eucharist frequently, even daily. These wishes of the church had been stated in the words of the Council of Trent:

> The holy council wishes indeed that at each Mass the faithful who are present should communicate, not only in spiritual desire, but sacramentally, by the actual reception of the Eucharist.[33]

In the same spirit, the encyclical set the first reception of communion at an earlier age.[34]

The papal document which came to serve as the theological basis for the various liturgical reforms was Pope Pius XII's *Mystici Corporis, The Mystical Body of Christ* (June 29, 1943). It highlighted the dignity of each member of the church as a member of the mystical body of Christ:

> Recognize, O Christian, your dignity, and being made a sharer of the divine nature go not back to your former worthlessness. . . . Keep in mind of what Head and of what Body you are a member.

Such membership binds the people together as one. The Mass gives special evidence "of our union among ourselves and with our divine

---

31. R. Kevin Seasoltz, *The New Liturgy: A Documentation, 1903-1965* (New York: Herder and Herder, 1966), XXVIII.

32. Pope St. Pius X, "The Restoration of Church Music," in *The New Liturgy: A Documentation, 1903-1965*, R. Kevin Seasoltz (New York: Herder and Herder, 1966), 3-4.

33. Sacred Congregation of the Council, "The Daily Reception of Holy Communion," in *The New Liturgy: A Documentation, 1903-1965*, R. Kevin Seasoltz (New York: Herder and Herder, 1966), 11.

34. Ibid., 14.

Head, marvelous as it is and beyond all praise."[35] This dignity and unity calls for the rightful place of the laity in worship.

These concepts were further developed and confirmed by Pius XII in *Mediator Dei*, (November 20, 1947). Intepreting and approving of the results of the work of the liturgical reform movement, the document states:

> By the waters of baptism, as by common right, Christians are made members of the mystical body of Christ the Priest, and by the "character" which is imprinted on their souls they are appointed to give worship to God; thus they participate, according to their condition, in the priesthood of Christ.[36]

This encyclical encouraged those desiring to reform the Mass. It has relevance for those active in church ministries today, including anyone appointed as special minister of communion to the sick.

To encourage participation, Pope Pius XII modified the Eucharistic fast. In *Christus Dominus, Apostolic Constitution* (January 6, 1953), he decreed that ordinary water does not break the Eucharistic fast. However, the midnight food fast remained. The sick are accommodated with special provisions:

> The sick, even though not confined to bed, may with the prudent advice of a confessor take something by way of drink or of true medicine exclusive of alcoholics."[37]

Pius XII further modified the fast in *Sacram Communionem* (March 19, 1957). A three-hour fast from food and alcoholic beverages and a one-hour fast from nonalcoholic beverages was established as the ordinary rule for all.[38] The provisions for the sick were also modified:

> The sick, even though not confined to bed, can take nonalcoholic drink and true and proper medicines, either liquid or solid, without limitation of time before celebrating Mass or receiving holy communion.[39]

---

35. Pope Pius XII, "The Mystical Body of Christ," in *The New Liturgy: A Documentation, 1903-1965*, R. Kevin Seasoltz (New York: Herder and Herder, 1966), 65, 81.

36. Seasoltz (ed), 88.

37. Pope Pius XII, "Christus Dominus," in *The New Liturgy: A Documentation, 1903-1965*, R. Kevin Seasoltz (New York: Herder and Herder, 1966), 183.

38. Pope Pius XII, "Sacram Communionem," in *The New Liturgy: A Documentation, 1903-1965*, R. Kevin Seasoltz (New York: Herder and Herder, 1966), 249.

39. Ibid., 250.

Finally, Pope Paul VI in *Sul Digiuno Eucharistico* (December 4, 1964) reduced the period of fasting from food and drink to one hour before communion.[40] This gesture shows the desire of the church to have the faithful partake at the table of the Lord.

The publication of the *Constitution on the Sacred Liturgy* (December 4, 1963) brought together the efforts of the reform movement in liturgy. The Council Fathers once more brought out the key notion of participation in the liturgy (CSL 14). They likewise underscored the communal nature of the liturgy (CSL 7). Finally, the document indicated that not only the priest, but also lay people, may have liturgical functions to perform:

> In liturgical celebrations each one, minister or layperson, who has an office to perform should do all of, but only, those parts which pertain to that office by the nature of the rite and the principles of liturgy (CSL 28).

Following the principles of reform in the *Constitution on the Sacred Liturgy*, all the rituals were revised. For example, *The Concelebration of Mass and Communion Under Both Kinds* (May 7, 1965) provided communion under both species for the assembly.[41] Nevertheless, neither the *Constitution on the Sacred Liturgy* nor The *Celebration of Mass and Communion Under Both Kinds* addressed the issue of lay ministers of Eucharist.

As a consequence of the Eucharistic reforms the number of communicants multiplied, while at the same time the availability of ordinary ministers (priests and deacons) diminished. Pope Paul VI responded in January, 1973 with *Immensae Caritatis*, known more formally as *Instruction on Facilitating Sacramental Communion in Particular Circumstances*. He stated: "First of all, provision must be made lest reception of Communion become impossible or difficult because of insufficient ministers."[42]

This lack of sufficient ministers could occur either during or outside of Mass. *Immensae Caritatis* names some pastoral situations: when the numbers of communicants at Mass is particularly large; when there is

---

40. Pope Paul VI, "Sul Digiuno Eucharistico," in *The New Liturgy: A Documentation, 1903-1965,* R. Kevin Seasoltz, (New York: Herder and Herder, 1966), 544.

41. Sacred Congregation of Rites, "The Concelebration of Mass and Communion Under Both Kinds," in *The New Liturgy: A Documentation, 1903-1965* R. Kevin Seasoltz (New York: Herder and Herder, 1966), 4-8.

42. Sacred Congregation for the Discipline of the Sacraments, "Instruction on Facilitating Sacramental Communion in Particular Circumstances," in *Vatican Council II: The Conciliar and Post Conciliar Documents,* Vol. 1, ed. Austin Flannery, O.P. (Northport: Costello Publishing Company, 1990), 226.

a need for a number of Eucharistic ministers to care for the sick; and when there is a grave emergency; for example, viaticum for a person in proximate danger of death. The document adds:

> Therefore, in order that the faithful . . . may not be deprived of this sacramental help and consolation, it has seemed appropriate to the Holy Father to establish extraordinary ministers, who may give Holy Communion to themselves and to other faithful . . .[43]

The description of the ministers for this Eucharistic ministry is noted in the document:

> The person who has been appointed to be an extraordinary minister of Holy Communion is necessarily to be duly instructed and should distinguish himself (sic) by his Christian life, faith, and morals. Let him strive to be worthy of this great office; . . . cultivate devotion to the Holy Eucharist; and show . . . reverence for the most holy Sacrament of the altar. Let no one be chosen whose selection may cause scandal among the faithful.[44]

In meeting the pastoral need for sufficient communion ministers, the document restores customs from the past. Once again, lay ministers distribute Eucharist. Once again, "the Sacred Host is placed in the hands of the communicant" by these ministers.[45]

Shortly following *Immensae Caritatis*, another document, *Holy Communion and Worship of the Eucharist Outside of Mass*, was published.[46] It reflected the official approval and development of special or lay ministers for communion. It provided rituals for the administration of communion and viaticum by an extraordinary minister.

In the 1982 revision of *Pastoral Care of the Sick: Rites of Anointing and Viaticum*, the church has set forth the outreach to the sick and dying. Of these rites, *Communion of the Sick in Ordinary Circumstances* and *Communion of the Sick in a Hospital or Institution*[47] are rites at which the lay Eucharistic ministers preside.

---

43. Ibid., 226-227.

44. Ibid., 228.

45. Ibid., 231.

46. Congregation for Divine Worship, "Holy Communion and Worship of the Eucharist Outside of Mass," in *The Rites of the Catholic Church*, (New York: The Pueblo Publishing Company, 1990), 633-698.

47. Congregation for Divine Worship, "The Rite of Communion of the Sick in a Hospital or Institution," 92-96, in *The Rites of the Catholic Church*, (New York: The Pueblo Publishing Company, 1990), 811-813.

In conclusion, these historical findings reveal the relationship of the two parallel trends of the Eucharistic practices of the church. When the early church practice of lay Eucharistic participation waned, so did the custom of lay persons taking communion to the sick. Conversely, the efforts of Vatican II to restore the participation of the assembly led to the restoration of the laity taking communion to the sick. The restoration of the early church tradition also restored the understanding of early Christian worship which grounds our current understanding of ministry to the sick.

The first Christians understood that they as community carried out the action of Eucharist. They believed partaking of communion was integral to the breaking of bread. It united the members of the assembly with Christ and with one another. To incorporate the absent, sick members of the community into this unity of the worshipping assembly, ministers in the name of the assembly took communion to them. *The Introduction of Pastoral Care to the Sick: Rites of Anointing and Viaticum* indicates this same understanding in the present practice of taking communion to the sick:

> Because the sick are prevented from celebrating the Eucharist with the rest of the community, the most important visits are those during which they receive holy communion. In receiving the body and blood of Christ, the sick are united sacramentally to the Lord and are reunited with the Eucharistic community from which illness has separated them (PCS 51).

One group in particular that suffers exclusion from the wider society, and often from the Eucharistic community, is the group comprised of people with HIV and AIDS. Eucharistic ministers will need an extra measure of sensitivity when ministering to people with HIV and AIDS because of the stigma and fear still attached to the disease in so many places.[48]

---

48. Further information may be found in an unpublished thesis by Mary McCue, *A Catechesis for Eucharistic Ministers Who Serve Persons with AIDS,* Santa Clara University, Santa Clara, CA, 1990.

TWO

Analysis of *The Rite of Communion of the Sick*

The collection of the official rituals of the church used in its care of the sick and the dying is called *Pastoral Care of the Sick: Rites of Anointing and Viaticum*. These rites were approved by the Conference of Catholic Bishops (November 18, 1982) and confirmed by the decree of the Sacred Congregation for the *Sacraments and Divine Worship* (December 11, 1982). The conference of bishops established November 27, 1983 as the mandatory effective date of these revised rites to be used in celebrations for the sick and the dying.[1] Usually, these rites are referred to as, simply, *Pastoral Care of the Sick*.

In *And You Visited Me: Sacramental Ministry to the Sick and the Dying*, Charles W. Gusmer,[2] contends that the most striking aspect of *Pastoral Care of the Sick* is its pastoral dimension. According to Gusmer, this emphasis is reflected in three ways. First, pastoral ministry to the sick is not the sole responsibility of the pastor. Rather, it involves the entire Christian Community. *Pastoral Care of the Sick* states: "This ministry is the common responsibility of all Christians, who should visit the sick, remember them in prayer, and celebrate the sacraments with them" (PCS 43). Second, these rites are meant to maintain the communal nature of the liturgical celebrations of the church. "Like the other sacraments, these too have a community aspect, which should be brought out as much as possible when they are celebrated" (Gen. Intro. 33). Third, pastoral adaptation was considered in the arrangement of the rites. The ordinary or normative rite is that which is celebrated in its full form

---

1. Decree of the National Conference of Catholic Bishops, *The Rites of the Catholic Church*, (New York: The Pueblo Publishing Company, 1990), 775.
2. Gusmer, x-xii, 53.

18 \ *Eucharistic Ministry to the Sick*

with the sick or the dying person and a community of believers. Yet, the rites accommodate the special circumstances of the sick and dying.

Indicative of this pastoral dimension, *Pastoral Care of the Sick* has two major divisions:

> The rites in Part I . . . are used by the Church to comfort the sick in time of anxiety, to encourage them to fight against illness, and perhaps to restore them to health (PCS 42). The rites in Part II . . . are used by the Church to comfort and strengthen a Christian in the passage from this life. The ministry to the dying places emphasis on trust in the Lord's promise of eternal life . . . (PCS 161).

Part I contains visits to the sick, communion to the sick, and the anointing of the sick. Part II contains the celebration of viaticum, commendation of the dying, prayers for the dead, and rites for exceptional circumstances. This division embodies the reforms authorized by Vatican II. Communion and anointing of the sick are the fundamental sacraments of the sick. Viaticum is the sacrament of the dying.[3]

The Rite of Communion of the Sick in Ordinary Circumstances,[4] which is chapter three of *Pastoral Care of the Sick*, provides for communion to the sick in the context of a liturgy of the word. It includes: the introductory rites of greeting, sprinkling with holy water and penitential rite; the liturgy of the word with reading, response, and general intercessions; the liturgy of communion with the Lord's prayer, communion, silent prayer, and prayer after communion; and the concluding rite.

Being familiar with and reflecting on the ritual and the prayer texts of this rite is an important part of eucharistic ministry to the sick. It prepares the minister to preside. The rite encourages catechesis:

> It is important that all the faithful, and above all the sick, be aided by suitable catechesis in preparing for and participating in the sacraments . . . especially if the celebration is to be carried out communally. . . . Understanding more, . . . the celebration of these sacraments will nourish, strengthen, and manifest faith more effectively. For the prayer of faith which accompanies the celebration of the sacrament is nourished by the profession of this faith (Gen. Intro. 36).

---

3. *Commentary: Pastoral Care of the Sick* (Washington, D.C.: United States Catholic Conference, 1983), 3.

4. In this chapter, *The Rite of Communion of the Sick in Ordinary Circumstances* will be referred to as *Communion of the Sick*.

Such liturgical catechesis of the minister is based on the rite at which she or he will preside. The following analysis of *Communion of the Sick* will focus on its ritual components: the symbolic action, the prayer texts, and the specific lectionary of the rite. The analysis of each ritual component will include: a description of the component, the method of analysis,[5] the summation of the analysis, and a conclusion that addresses how the analysis helps shape the preparation of the ministers.

I. The Symbolic Action of Rite of *Communion of the Sick*

What is symbolic action? It is the action of the assembled community expressing faith and participating in its mystery, the Paschal Mystery of Jesus Christ. The Eucharist relates to the events of the life, death, and resurrection of Jesus Christ which gave rise to the Christian community. In the ritual action, the community expresses and "represents" the religious experience of the Christ event. It does so through the human actions of gathering, listening, sharing the bread, and departing. The dynamic of these actions is the Holy Spirit. The celebration enables the community to share in the life of Christ.[6]

Rites of communion outside of Mass are "perceived and celebrated as continuations of the community's liturgical action in the Eucharist."[7] Therefore, the rite of *Communion of the Sick* is the continuation of the Eucharistic action of the Sunday assembly. In taking communion to the "faithful who are deprived of their rightful and accustomed place in the Eucharistic community" (RCS 73), the eucharistic minister is instrumental in extending the action of the Sunday assembly. Thus, the sick are incorporated into the action of the full Eucharistic assembly.[8]

The Eucharistic minister brings communion to the sick in the context of a liturgical rite, *Communion of the Sick*. As representative of the full assembly, the Eucharistic minister presides at this liturgy. Because this rite is the continuation of the community's liturgical action of eucha-

---

5. Rita Claire Dorner, O.P., "Method of Analyzing a Liturgical Rite," from lecture, Santa Clara University (April 2, 1992).
6. Dallen, 16-18.
7. Mitchell, 249.
8. Ibid., 255.

rist, it is consciously modeled on the unitive liturgies of word and table.[9] Thus, the rite calls for similar actions; the four symbolic actions are gathering as community, listening to the Word, sharing Bread, and being blessed. In the following analysis, each symbolic action will be considered in its human, biblical, and ecclesial settings.

1. Gathering as Community

Human Setting

To gather is an integral activity of the human condition. A diversity of people come together for a common purpose. Gathering to do a specific action unifies the individuals into a definite group. People come together for a variety of reasons: to learn, to work, to celebrate, to recreate, to give honor, and to reach out in support. Learning is the basis of numerous educational gatherings of people: classes in schools and universities, groups attending conventions and workshops, and self-help groups. An individual's job immediately places that person within the work community of a company or institution. People gather to celebrate special occasions of life: birthdays, anniversaries, weddings, graduations, and other achievements. Recreation brings the gathered crowd to theaters, sport arenas, resorts, and fairs. People gather at parades honoring special events or persons. Groups unite to demonstrate support for causes. The community of neighbors supports families who have lost members in death or individuals who are sick.

Biblical Setting

Biblical gatherings reflect motivations similar to those above. Many instances of people gathering to learn from the Teacher are noted in Christian Scriptures. The following citings illustrate this: "... word got around that Jesus was home. At that they began to gather in great numbers. . . . he was delivering God's word to them . . ." (Mk. 2:1-2). "The crowds went in search of Jesus . . . They were spellbound by his teaching . . ." (Lk. 4:32, 42). Groups celebrated: ". . . there was a wedding at Cana in Galilee, and the mother of Jesus was there. Jesus and his disciples had likewise been invited to the celebration" (Jn. 2:1). His followers honored Jesus: ". . . as Jesus rode along seated on the colt, many spread their garments on the road . . ." (Mk. 11:7-8). "The whole

---

9. Ibid., 249.

multitude of the disciples began to rejoice and praise God . . . 'Blessed is the King who comes in the name of the Lord' (Lk. 19:37). Finally, support during difficult times is evidenced in Scripture: ". . . a dead man was being carried out, the only son of a widowed mother of Naim. A considerable crowd of townsfolk were with her" (Lk. 7:13). "A large crowd of people . . . to be healed of their diseases . . . to be cured of unclean spirits. . . . the whole crowd was trying to touch Jesus because power went out from him which cured all" (Lk. 6:17-19).

Ecclesial Setting

James Dallen indicates the impetus for liturgical gathering is the same as that for human and biblical gatherings: gathering "implies an interaction through which unified and purposeful activity will be possible."[10] The liturgical action of gathering involves people becoming aware of one another and realizing that together they form a celebrating community. Through hospitable, welcoming interaction, the assembly prepares for a unified and purposeful listening and sharing.[11]

In gathering for the liturgy of the sick, the hospitable, welcoming interaction takes place among the sick, the minister, the family, and friends. The introductory rites of *Communion of the Sick* foster the unity of this community. These rites bring people "into the presence of God through an awareness of themselves as the gathered People of God."[12] The greeting, "The Lord be with you," is a prayer of the presider that the sick and those gathered are indeed experiencing being present together before the Lord. The presence of the representative from the parish celebration of Eucharist unites the sick to the worshipping community from which they are separated. The sprinkling rite reminds the faith community that they are united with Christ and one another. Finally, the penitential rite calls people to a remembrance of God's mercy. The litany, "Lord, Have Mercy," expresses the sense of the community being in the presence of the Lord.

---

10. Dallen, 28.
11. Ibid., 31.
12. Ibid., 32.

2. Listening to the Word

Human Setting

Storytelling is inherent to human living. Human lives create the story content. Sharing a story enables its continuance. Further, reflection on a story makes possible its influence on the teller and listeners alike. Circumstances of life shape the unique stories of individuals. Yet, the story of an individual can also shape circumstances, can touch the lives of others.

Telling and hearing stories happens in the midst of a gathered people. Stories are related at the various gatherings noted earlier. Students learn by listening to stories. Professors teach by telling stories. Stories flow among the people at work. When a community gathers to celebrate a birthday or anniversary, it celebrates the story of birth or wedding; the telling of and listening to stories fill the festivities. Sometimes people gather just to share stories, to spend time remembering. At other times, they gather with those in need, such as the sick. The community supports the sick by compassionately listening to their stories. Listening to stories of heroes or departed loved ones enables those people to live on among us. Thus, to share stories is the human way to communicate.

Biblical Setting

In the biblical setting, Jesus listened to the stories of those in the community. As a boy of 12, he remained "in the temple sitting in the midst of the teachers, listening to them and asking them questions. All who heard him were amazed at his intelligence and answers" (Lk. 2:46-47). Jesus also listened to the human stories of need. For example, he listened to the Canaanite woman: "Lord, Son of David, have pity on me! My daughter is terribly troubled by a demon. . . . Help me, Lord. . . . Please, Lord, . . . even the dogs eat the leavings that fall from their master's tables" (Mt. 15:22-27).

Jesus listened to Jairus, who fell at his feet, "earnestly" telling his story: "My little daughter is critically ill. Please come and lay your hands on her so that she may get well and live" (Mk. 5:22-23). Jesus was attentive to the poor, hungry, sick, blind, lame, deaf, paralyzed, and mentally ill found throughout the Christian Scriptures.

As well as listening to their stories, Jesus told stories of his own to the crowds and his disciples. The use of parable, a metaphorical story form, enabled Jesus to unveil the mystery of God and God's kingdom and to involve his listeners.[13] Using the face of nature or common life in simile, Jesus invited his listeners to new thoughts about God. In telling such open-ended stories, Jesus called the listeners to response, to conversion.[14] On one such occasion, a crowd gathered around him. . . . He began to instruct them . . . by the use of parables. . . . Listen carefully to this." Jesus told the parable of the seeds. The seeds that landed on the footpath, in rocky soil or into thornbushes bore no fruit. Only the seed that fell on good soil, took root and bore fruit. "The seed is the word." To the extent that the disciples of Jesus "listen to the word, take it to heart," they will "yield at thirty and sixty and a hundredfold" (Mk. 4:1-20).

Ecclesial Setting

James Dallen capsulizes the liturgical process of listening to the Word as community:

> The action of the gathered assembly listening together, the central focus of the Liturgy of the Word, directs the remembering and shapes the imagining. It recalls the pattern of God's relating to humanity and gives foundations to our hopes for the future. Our community's memory is presented in an objective form, and a rich store of images is recalled through the proclamation of the scriptures. This listening further . . . deepens our realization that we gather at God's call and that it is God's Word that creates us as a community.[15]

In celebrating the liturgy of the sick, the gathered community listens to scripture stories particular to the rite of *Communion of the Sick*. As Christ is present in the proclamation of the Word, listening to the Word is nourishment to the faith of the sick. A few moments of silent response to the Word allows time for the sick to relate their human story to the Word. A brief explanation of the reading by the minister or a shared reflection with those present will further enable connections between their story and God's story. Their story is part of God's relationship with them. The sick are invited beyond their human pain

---

13. Daniel J. Harrington, S.J., "The Gospel According to Mark," in *The New Jerome Biblical Commentary*, eds. Raymond E. Brown, S.S., Joseph Fitzmeyer, S.J. and Roland E. Murphy, O.Carm. (Englewood Cliffs: Prentice Hall, 1990), 605-606.

14. Philip Van Linden, C.M., "Mark," in *The Collegeville Bible Commentary*, eds. Dianne Bergant, C.S.A. and Robert J. Darris, O.F.M. (Collegeville: The Liturgical Press, 1989), 912.

15. Dallen, 33-34.

3. Sharing Bread

Human Setting

Sharing a meal is symbolic of the relationship among those present. In sharing food and drink, they also share who they are for one another. The sharing of food ranges from snacks at coffee break, hot dogs at sports events, popcorn at the movies, hors d'oeuvres at social events, full meals at the family table, and the festival food of special banquets.

When an individual is unable to eat at the family table because of sickness, food is taken to him or her. Usually a family member visits while the sick person eats. The bond of family is confirmed for the sick person. Preparing and sharing food with a sick friend or neighbor not only alleviates her physical hunger, but enables a celebration of an existing relationship.

Biblical Setting

Table fellowship is characteristic of the ministry of Jesus. The Gospels tell of the significant meals Jesus ate with friends, sinners, the hungry crowds, marginal people, wedding quests, and his disciples. For example, "while Jesus was at table in Matthew's home, many tax collectors and those known as sinners came to join Jesus and his disciples at dinner" (Mt. 9:10). "Jesus was in Bethany reclining at table in the house of Simon the leper . . ." (Mk. 14:3). "Jesus went to the Pharisee's home and reclined to eat" (Lk. 7:36). "Taking the five loaves and two fish, Jesus . . . blessed . . . broke the loaves, and gave them to the disciples to distribute to the hungry crowd" (Mt. 14:19; Mk. 8:7; 6:41; Lk. 9:16; Jn. 6:11). The one meal that symbolized all the meals that Jesus shared was the Last Supper. This meal was different from the others. Jesus made the sharing of the bread and the cup synonymous with his life. "During the meal Jesus took bread, blessed it, broke it, and gave it to his disciples. . . . this is my body. . . . Then he took the cup, gave thanks and gave it to them. . . . this is my blood" (Mt. 26:26-28).

to the hope their faith offers in the acceptance of God in their lives. In intercessions, the community asks God to help the sick live out the Word and deal with the problems and needs of the sick.

Ecclesial Setting

The sharing of bread and cup in the Liturgy of the Eucharist follows the ritual of Jesus' table fellowship at his last supper. The assembly presents food and drink to be shared, joins in blessing God, breaks the bread, and shares the holy gifts. In this case, the pattern of sharing, concern, care, responsibility, and solidarity which characterize the gathering and listening now grows stronger and becomes clearer as the assembly models its activity on what Jesus did. The assembly's memory is enlivened as its experience of God in Christ is brought into the present. And, if the interaction and exchange among the assembly is indeed patterned on Jesus' activity, the imagination is filled. We are given a taste of the kingdom.[16]

Celebrating the rite of *Communion of the Sick* is continuing the Eucharistic action of the Sunday assembly. In the Communion rite, the sick and those assembled receive the Bread blessed and broken at the full eucharistic celebration. The sick are united sacramentally to Christ and reunited to the worshipping community. "Taking communion to the sick from the community's Eucharistic celebration" is a "symbol of unity between the community and its sick members" (RCS 73).

4. Being Blessed

Human Setting

To bless another is to express solicitude for his or her well-being. This care and concern usually takes the form of good wishes. Some common expressions are: "Have a good day;" "Wish you the best;" "Take care;" "Have a safe trip;" "Birthday blessings of happiness, health and many years of life;" "Wish you success;" "Congratulations;" "Get well soon;" "Be at peace;" "May you find comfort in your sorrow;" and "Good luck." Many blessings are expressed in the form of praise or thanks: "Your friendship is a blessing to me;" or "All your help is a blessing." Blessing is also given for gifts, especially for food at mealtime.

Usually such good wishes are accompanied with touch: joined hands, a grasp of the arm, a pat on the back, or a hug. The practice of sending greeting cards which cover every occasion of life expresses our thoughtful attentiveness to others. The cards convey the blessings we

---

16. Ibid., 36.

wish conferred on others. However expressed, blessing another is a form of prayer. We pray that a particular wish be granted.

Biblical Setting

The New Testament texts refer to Jesus blessing specific groups. Once, the people brought "their little children" to Jesus "to have him touch them. . . . He embraced them and blessed them, placing his hands on them" (Mk. 10:13,16). The greeting of the Risen Jesus, his wish for his frightened disciples, was: "Peace be with you" (Jn. 20:19). At his ascension, Jesus, "with hands upraised, blessed them. As he blessed, he left them . . . ." Filled "with joy," the disciples "praised God" (Lk. 24:50-53). Jesus also blessed food: "Taking the five loaves and two fishes, Jesus raised his eyes to heaven, pronounced a blessing . . ." (Mt. 14:19; Mk. 6:41; 8:7; Lk. 9:16; Jn. 6:11). Again, "during the meal Jesus took bread, blessed it . . . . Then he took the cup, gave thanks . . ." (Mt. 26:26-28).

Ecclesial Setting

The status of blessing within the Church is stated in the Decree of the *Book of Blessings:*

> The celebration of blessings holds a privileged place among all the sacramentals created by the Church for the pastoral benefit of the people of God. As a liturgical action, the celebration leads the faithful to praise God and prepares them for the principal effect of the sacraments. By celebrating a blessing the faithful can also sanctify various situations and events in their lives.[17]

Every blessing flows from God. Ministers of the church offer thanks in praise of God's name. They ask for divine blessings for other persons or the works of creation. Whoever blesses others in God's name invokes the divine help upon individuals or upon an assembled people.[18]

The celebration of the rite of *Communion of the Sick* concludes with a blessing of those assembled. Lay eucharistic ministers of the sick may preside at the blessing by virtue of their ministry and by use of the formularies designated for lay ministers.[19] In the blessing of the sick in this rite, the Eucharistic minister invokes God as Trinity, asking God's blessing and protection for the sick.

---

17. International Commission on English in the Liturgy, *Book of Blessings* (Collegeville: The Liturgical Press, 1989), xxi.

18. Ibid., Gen. Intro., 6.

19. Ibid., 18.

This analysis of the symbolic actions of the rite of *Communion of the Sick* helps shape the preparation of those preparing for Eucharistic ministry to the sick. Through reflection on the activity of the assembly, the ministers become aware of the structural dynamics of Christian worship. Worship is the activity of the liturgical assembly. Eucharist is an action done by the assembly. Specifically, this reflection enables an understanding of the purpose of the actions of the liturgy of *Communion of the Sick*. It also clarifies for the ministers that specific human experiences undergird the understanding of the *Communion of the Sick*.

Each of the symbolic actions of the rite of *Communion of the Sick* which continue the action of the full eucharistic assembly have a definite but interrelated purpose. The welcoming exchange of gathering, with the sick and others present, enables a unified listening and sharing. Listening to the Word recalls God's relating to humanity, especially to the sick, and gives the sick hope for the future. Our realization that we gather at God's call and that God's Word creates us as community deepens as we listen. Sharing the Eucharistic food is sharing a communal meal. Like listening, sharing communion enables our unity. The sick are united with Christ, with the Christian assembly, and with the full Eucharistic action. The liturgy concludes with the sick being blessed. The presider asks God to bless the sick in their need, to favor them with courage and protection.

An understanding of each of the actions of the liturgy, *Communion of the Sick*, in their human, biblical, and ecclesial setting is necessary in order to understand the whole liturgy. The social aspect of humanity engenders the gathering of a people for a specific activity. The telling of and listening to stories is the human way to communicate. The significance of food and drink is the nourishment of the people. Viewing the actions of the liturgy in the biblical setting affirms that Jesus accomplished his mission of salvation through human words and actions. In doing what Jesus did, the Church in its sacramental life continues to use those human actions significantly associated with the historical events of Jesus' salvific mission.

II. The Prayer Texts of the Rite of *Communion of the Sick*

This second part of the analysis of the rite of *Communion of the Sick* includes: the prayer texts, the dialogical exchanges, and the intercessions of the assembly. The dialogical exchanges are the exchanges between the presider and the sick or the assembly present. They are not addressed to God. The intercessions consist of the petitions of prayer of this assembly.

The theological meaning of the prayer texts is probed through an analysis of the images of the individual prayer texts. The method used to arrive at this meaning is to ask questions that enable an understanding of the underlying theology, Christology, ecclesiology, pneumatology, and anthropology. The questions are based on the images of

- God:
  To whom is the prayer addressed?
  How is God named?
  How is God described?
  What deeds of God are cited and proclaimed as the occasion for the prayer of the church?
- Christ:
  How is Jesus named?
  How is Jesus' relationship to the church described?
  Are there implicit or explicit references to the Paschal Mystery?
- Holy Spirit:
  How is the Holy Spirit named?
  What is the work of the Spirit on behalf of the church?
- Church:
  How does the church name itself?
  What petitions does the church ask for?
- People of the Assembly:
  How is the human person described?
  How is the assembly described?

The summation of the above questions draws from the analysis of the individual prayer texts and dialogical exchanges.

To whom is the prayer addressed?

Two of the eight prayer texts of the rite of *Communion of the Sick* are addressed to God. Three prayer texts are addressed to the community. Both God and community are addressed in three texts. More prayer texts address community than God. This seems to clearly indicate the communal nature of this rite. This means the rite is celebrated with a community. Communal also includes this reality: "In receiving the body

Analysis of The Rite of Communion of the Sick / 29

and blood of Christ, the sick are united sacramentally to the Lord and are reunited with the eucharistic community from which illness has separated them" (PCS 51).

How is God named?

The prayers invoke God as **God** (83A/90B/91B) three times. The other prayers name God as **Lord** (81A/86) twice and as **Our Father** (87A) and the trinitarian form, **the Father and the Son and the Holy Spirit** (91B), each once. These titles for God are indicative of the more traditional names given to God.

How is God described?

The descriptions of God within the prayer texts exhibit a more personal faith relationship with the sick. God is characterized as a God of **peace** (81A) and **mercy** (91B). These seem appropriate attributes for the God from whom the sick seek compassion and healing. The **almighty** (83A/91B), **all-powerful** (90B) **Father** (87A) conveys God's initiative to love, to reassure the sick of this love in their illness.

What deeds of God are cited and proclaimed as the occasion for prayer of the church?

God unfolds the mystery of God's love in great deeds in our regard. The specific deed of God found in the prayer texts of this rite is God's **nourishment** (90B) given through God's **holy gifts.** God gives strength through this food from heaven, the eucharist.

How is Jesus named?

This gift of eucharist (nourishment, healing and unity) is contingent on the saving actions of Jesus. These acts of redemption are encapsulated in the titles given to Jesus. To use the title **Lord Jesus** (83A/3 times), is significant. To believe that Jesus is Lord is to believe that he is risen and glorified at the right hand of the Father. He has won a decisive eschatological victory over the powers of evil. **Christ** (82-83A/88B), **Christ the Lord** (87A), **Lord** (83A/4 times;88B) and **Jesus the Christ** (90B) are also names given the Risen Jesus. The greatness of God's love shown in the salvific death of **God's Son** (91B) is poignantly demonstrated in referring to Jesus as the **Lamb of God** (88B).

How is Jesus' relationship to the church described?

The relationship of Jesus to the church is described implicitly. **Who by his death and resurrection has redeemed us** (82A) implies Jesus is the **Redeemer** of the People of God.

Are there implicit or explicit references to the Paschal Mystery?

Jesus continues to **nourish** (83A) and to **heal (88B).** Jesus acts through and in the Church. God's plan of salvation is symbolically mediated through the sacramental life of the church. Thus, the presence of Christ and his love is tangible in sacrament. His Paschal Mystery is celebrated in the symbolic actions of the church's liturgical prayer. The salvific effect of his **death and resurrection** (82A) is explicitly expressed in the prayer texts. It is through **this celebration** (83A/liturgy of the sick) that Jesus **takes away the sins of the world** (88B), **heals** and **brings us strength** (83A). In praying with Jesus as he **taught us to pray** (87A) to the Father, we express the hope of living a sacramental life in its fullness: may **your Kingdom come** (87A).

How is the Holy Spirit named?

The Holy Spirit is referred to only twice. The reference is to **your Spirit** (90B) and **Holy Spirit** (91B).

What is the work of the Spirit on behalf of the Church?

Since this liturgy of the sick is a continuation of the liturgical action of the full eucharistic celebration, the work of the Spirit is described in the celebration of eucharist. In the epiclesis of the eucharistic prayer we call on the power of the Spirit. **Let your Spirit come upon these gifts to make them holy, so that they may become for us the body and blood of our Lord, Jesus Christ.** We also pray that **we who share** in the Lord may **be brought together in unity by the Holy Spirit** (EP II). We recall these works of the Holy Spirit in the texts of this rite when we **thank the all powerful God** for nourishing us (the sick) **through your holy** gifts (90B). Further, we ask God to **pour out your Spirit upon us** and to give us **the strength of this food from heaven** (90B).

How does the church name itself?

You (81A) refers to the **sick person** and others present at the liturgy of *Communion of the Sick*. The community is addressed as **brothers and sisters** (83A). The assembled as **needy** is indicated in the Our Father: **give us our daily bread** (87A). In asking for **mercy on us** (83A), **us** speaks to the sick and others as **sinners.** The implication of **sinners** is expressed in a variety of forms: **forgive us** (83A); **forgive us . . . as we forgive** (87A); and, always potential sinners, **lead us not into temptation but deliver us from evil** (87A). Yet, **happy are we who are called to the Lord's supper** (88B). We are the **redeemed** (82A). We **call to mind our baptism into Christ, who by his death and resurrection has redeemed us** (82A). As Church, a redeemed sinful People, the sick are united in and through Christ. In sharing eucharist, the sick celebrate and participate in the paschal mystery of Christ through the dynamic of the Spirit, hopeful of future glory.

What petitions does the church ask for?

The longer list of petitions sought in the prayer texts seems indicative of our need before God. More specifically, we realize that the Spirit of Christ has power to transform us. The intercessions expressed are: **have mercy** (83A/6 times); **forgive us** (83A), **only say the word and I will be healed** (88B); **pour out your Spirit on us** (90B); **keep us single-minded in your service** through **the strength of this food** (90B); and, **bless us and protect us** (91B). Along with these, we have the seven petitions of Jesus in the Our Father. Within the prayer text of *Communion of the Sick*, these petitions have striking relational and healing tones.

How is the human person described?

In prayer text 88B, the sick and those present refer to themselves as individuals: **I am not worthy to receive you, . . . say the word and I shall be healed.** This only reference to the individual is significant. The prayer texts bring out the communal aspect of *Communion to the Sick*. The liturgy incorporates the sick into the full Eucharistic community.

In conclusion, reflection on the prayer texts and dialogical exchanges in *Communion of the Sick* is the basis for catechesis of the Eucharistic ministers. Study of these texts enables understanding of the liturgy of the sick from another perspective. The prayer texts and dialogical exchanges support and inform the symbolic actions of the assembly. The actions of the assembly celebrate the mystery of our faith.

The study of the individual prayer texts gives the eucharistic ministers the opportunity to clarify their understanding of the beliefs particular to this liturgy of the sick. The ministers, in turn, are able to reflect the meaning of the celebration to the sick. Briefly, the prayers reflect: God is Trinity, model of communal love. It is God's initiative to love the sick, to nourish them with the Bread of Life. Jesus concretized God's love in human form. As Redeemer, the Risen Jesus heals, strengthens, and gives hope to the sick. As members of the People of God, the sick are united to Christ and to the community when they partake of the food from the common table.

III. The Lectionary of the Rite of *Communion of the Sick*

This final part of the analysis reflects on the lectionary specific to the rite of *Communion of the Sick*. The rite provides a selection of five readings, including gospel texts from John: 6:51, 6:54-58, 14:6, and 15:5, and a fifth lection from the first letter of John, 4:16.[20] These texts will be the focus of the lectionary analysis.

The above lections will be analyzed by identifying the following elements in each pericope: the literary form; reference to the symbolic action of the rite; the images of God (Father), Jesus, and Holy Spirit; the relationship of these images to the person or persons doing the rite; and, the theme of the reading.

The summation of each of the above elements draws from the data of the analysis of these readings from the liturgy of the Word.

---

20. An appropriate reading from Part III of *Pastoral Care of the Sick*, "Readings, Responses, and Verses from Sacred Scripture," may be used in place of those cited. See PCS 297.

The Literary Form

Three of the gospel lections are in the form of a discourse. John 6:51 and 6:54-58 are selections from the discourse of Jesus as **bread of life.** John 14:6 is part of the farewell discourse of Jesus. John 15:5 is taken from the metaphor of the vine and the branches. 1 John 4:16 is an apostolic teaching.

Reference to the Symbol of Sharing Nourishment

The discourse on the bread of life (Jn. 6: 25-59) connotes two levels of meaning. Both the meanings as well as the shift of meaning are found in verse 51. **I myself am the living bread come down from heaven** (v. 51a) refers to Jesus as revealer of the Father. This is the topic of the first part of the discourse. The topic shifts to specifying the bread that Jesus gives in Eucharistic terms: **the bread I will give is my flesh, for the life of the world** (v. 51b).[21] Verses 53-56 expand this idea about bread as Jesus' flesh: my flesh is real food and my blood real drink (v 56). The vine and the branches imagery (Jn. 15:5) is symbolic of this Eucharistic nourishment. It is linked to the teaching of the necessity of remaining with Jesus.[22] For a Eucharistic people, Jesus is the way, and **the truth, and the life** (Jn. 14:6). Jesus is the source of life and truth.

Images of God

The one who renews and refreshes is named **God.** God is also imaged as **Father** and **Love.** Jesus is referred to as Jesus four times. Images for Jesus are: **living bread from heaven; bread from heaven; the way, the truth, and the life;** and **the vine.** Jesus imaged as gift of life, nourishment, and strength corresponds to the needs of the sick.

Relationship of These Images to the Sick

The Father sent the Son to give life. The life of the Son is the Father's own life. Jesus extends this type of relationship to the sick when they

---

21. Pheme Perkins, "The Gospel According to John," in *The New Jerome Biblical Commentary*, eds. Raymond E. Brown, S.S., Joseph Fitzmyer, S.J. and Roland E. Murphy, O.Carm. (Englewood Cliffs: Prentice Hall, 1990), 962.
22. Ibid., 976.

partake of the **bread from heaven.**[23] As the source of **life** and **truth,** Jesus is their link to the Father. The image of the **vine and branches** reflects the unity between Christ and the sick: **the one who remains in me and I in him [her] bears much fruit.** In Christ, the human pain and suffering of the sick become redemptive (PCS 3). In Christ, the sick are united to the worshipping community. Sharing Eucharist is also a pledge of **life eternal.**

The Themes of the Lections

The core thought of each lection is that:
Jesus is the Bread of Life (Jn. 6:51).
Whoever eats this bread has eternal life (Jn. 6:54-58).
All come to the Father through Jesus (Jn. 14:6).
To remain in Jesus is to bear much fruit (Jn. 15:5).
God is love (1 Jn. 4:16).

As the Bread of Life, Jesus is the sacramental nourishment of the sick. The presence of the Spirit-filled, risen Jesus enables the sick to strengthen their faith and renew their hope. Peace in their situation of sickness is possible.

In conclusion, reflection on the lections for the rite of *Communion of the Sick* complements the study of the symbolic action and the prayer texts as the basis for catechesis of Eucharistic ministers preparing to take communion to the sick. Pondering the scriptures used in the liturgy of the Word enables the minister to proclaim the Word to the sick in their present human experience.

God's Word must be broken open in faith by the minister. It is not enough for the minister to believe in his or her heart. The sick must be able to perceive the minister's faith in what he or she does and says in carrying out the ministry of the Word.

The minister helps the sick to make connections between their personal story and the story of God in the proclaimed Word. Their story is part of God's relationship with them. The minister encourages the sick to accept the invitation of the Word to go beyond their human pain to the hope their faith offers in the acceptance of God in their lives.

---

23. Ibid., 962.

THREE

A Catechetical Process for Preparing Ministers to the Sick

Introduction

These liturgical catechetical sessions are for eucharistic ministers preparing to take communion to the sick. The presumption is that participants have completed catechesis in preparation to serve as ministers of Eucharist, and that they have also been so commissioned. This catechesis enables the participants to preside at the rite of communion to the sick. The process includes reflecting on the theology of the rite which gives understanding to lived faith. It also affords familiarity with *The Rite of Communion of the Sick in Ordinary Circumstances* (Rite 71-91), which ensures a focused and prayerful celebration of the liturgy with the sick.

The communal nature of the Church's liturgical celebrations influenced the composition of all of the rites included in *Pastoral Care of the Sick: Rites of Anointing and Viaticum.* Commentary for the rites states: "As celebrations of, for, and by the Church, the sacraments are best understood and experienced when celebrated in their most complete form with a community of Christian believers."[1] This principle applies strongly to the Church's ministry to the sick. Sickness isolates a person from the celebrating Eucharistic community. Therefore, the community reaches out to the sick. The rite emphasizes taking communion to the sick as the "symbol of unity" between the community of the Eucharistic assembly and its sick members (RCS 73). This proposed catechesis advocates communion to the sick within the context of liturgy of the word with a community, thus maintaining "full and communal celebration."[2]

---

1. From ICEL Newsletter, (April-June, 1983) Washington D.C., 4.
2. Ibid., 5.

The Eucharistic ministers approved for this service of communion to the sick meet for four consecutive weeks. This liturgical catechesis takes place in a suitable parish meeting room. The four sessions are based on the the structure of the rite:

1. The Community Reaches Out in Compassion,
2. The Community Listens and Responds in Faith,
3. The Community Unites in Celebrative Sharing,
4. The Community Reflects and Prays Together.

Each catechetical session provides opportunity for the participants to experience: welcoming into community, gathering prayer, sharing life experience and faith reflection, becoming aware of serving justly, and participating in ritual prayer. The ministers will also practice the skills involved in ministry to the sick.

This plan is a liturgical catechesis because it "strengthens faith and summons Christians to conversion" by preparing them "for full and active participation in the liturgy."[3] This catechesis is based on the human lives of the people. It relates the experience of sickness to the liturgy of the sick.

Liturgical catechesis approaches this task of preparation through reflection on the human experience of sickness, the scripture lectionary for the rite, the rite itself, and the Christology set forth in the rite. Participants examine the human experience of sickness which the liturgy of the sick addresses. Catechesis prepares the ministers to proclaim the Word of God to the sick. The Word interprets the human experience of sickness. Participants reflect on the rite by exploring the power of the symbolic gestures, actions, and words of the praying community. In catechesis, the ministers reflect on the power of the Paschal Mystery of Christ present in the liturgical community. Along with these ritual components, liturgical catechesis incorporates the elements of building community, sharing stories and beliefs, and participating in just service.[4] In this way, the ministers prepare to preside at the liturgy of the sick and the sick will be reunited to the full eucharistic assembly through the celebration of the liturgy.

---

3. National Conference of Catholic Bishops, *Sharing the Light of Faith: National Catechetical Directory for Catholics of the United States* (Washington, D.C.: United States Catholic Conference, 1978), 113.

4. Rita Claire Dorner, O.P., from lecture, Santa Clara University, (April 2, 1992).

Session One:
The Community Reaches Out in Compassion

Catechist Reflection

Ministry to the sick embraces people broken with sickness. Knowledge of the effects of human sickness informs the manner of approach to the sick. Sickness, according to Charles Gusmer,[5] is representative of a crisis situation in the life of the person who is ill. The crisis is in communication with oneself, others, and the church.

In the crisis of communication with oneself, the human body is no longer experienced as an extension of one's inner being. Instead, it becomes an object to be exposed, probed, and manipulated by all who provide care. There is also the temporal disability of wondering, "When will I get better?"

Within this crisis of communication with oneself, Gusmer sees a correlation of Kubler-Ross' stages of dying and the stages of serious illness. The initial period is that of silence. The sick do not wish to talk. They are totally taken up with sickness. In the period of aggression, the sick lash out at their milieu. The perception is that family and friends visit seldom, the medical staff is incompetent, and even the church neglects them. This is really not a personal affront but a cry for help, for love and understanding, for a simple personal presence. The period of depression is a fruitful time for interiorization. The sick take stock of the situation and themselves. Rebirth can follow. The final period is acceptance. The affliction is either endured with serenity or met with contempt.

A second crisis of communication with others happens because normal life is disrupted. Sickness usually isolates the sick person from family, work or profession, circle of friends, those things and relationships that make life most worth living.

The third crisis of communication is with the church. This is a common experience for those Christians who were active in their parish and now feel forgotten. To cope with all the effects of sickness, the sick need help and support.

Those with HIV and AIDS require a special measure of compassionate support. Alongside the physical pain associated with the disease's devastating toll, those with AIDS often experience intense emotional suffering. Feelings of guilt and shame, commonly associated

---

5. Gusmer, 139-142.

38 \ *Eucharistic Ministry to the Sick*

with serious illness in general, may be intensified in the case of the person with HIV or AIDS.

If the person with HIV or AIDS is gay, social retribution and homophobia, as well as internalized shame, often takes a toll. For some, the diagnosis of AIDS necessitates the decision of whether or not to disclose for the first time their emotional/sexual orientation to family members. Thus they face communicating simultaneously the reality of their impending death and their sexual identity. They run the risk of being rejected by significant persons in their lives at the very time they need much support and affirmation.

Those who have contracted the disease through intravenous drug use experience their own measure of shame and marginalization. In such cases, there is the tendency on the part of many to see AIDS as a moral rather than a medical issue; as a judgment or punishment rather than as a disease.

The physical and emotional suffering of advanced cases of AIDS is interwoven with an overwhelming experience of loss, made more poignant by the comparative youth of many of those who die of AIDS. The average age of persons with AIDS is about 36 years, an age when one expects to be highly independent and productive.

The anguish that a person with AIDS undergoes on the journey to death can attack and erode spiritual health. The sick person must deal with doubts and fears regarding his or her own worth as a person. Feelings of grief, isolation, and loneliness may become overwhelming. This human state of brokenness calls out for the witness of compassionate presence.[6]

The ability to reach out to those in pain flows from the experience of being human. To be human is to learn to weep, to keep vigil, to wait for the dawn. To be compassionate is "to grieve, to experience sorrow, to cry out with."[7] Compassion is difficult. It exacts the inner disposition "to go with others to the place where they are weak, vulnerable, lonely and broken."[8] The initial response to suffering is either to want to "fix it" or not to want to be involved. Compassion takes another route – it requires "being one with" the suffering person, entering into his or her

---

6. For a further description of AIDS see an unpublished thesis by Mary McCue, *A Catechesis for Eucharistic Ministers Who Serve Persons with AIDS,* Santa Clara University, Santa Clara, CA, 1990.

7. Henri J.M. Nouwen, *Out of Solitude* (Notre Dame: Ave Maria Press, 1975), 34.

8. Henri J.M. Nouwen, *The Way of the Heart* (New York: Ballintine Books, 1985), 20.

pain. Personal presence in this stance is a healing presence, is compassion.

Genuine compassion is exemplified in this story of the encounter of a sick woman and a visiting minister:

> The patient just sobbed. What could I say? Words seemed to intensify the tears. A phrase came to mind, "Create silence." That seemed to be the wisdom for the moment. She clutched my hand. The silence was punctuated by her sobs. Finally, they became fewer and farther between, then they ceased with a sigh. "Thank you," she said gratefully. "I needed someone to let me cry." That time created trust between us and we later had many long visits when we talked about God's presence in her life.[9]

Such compassion combats the isolation caused by the suffering and loneliness of sickness. Hearts begin to open to each other. Community is possible. Concrete, tangible care assures connectedness to the community.

The gospel stories point to compassion as the basis of Jesus' earthly ministry. In his words, his mission is to "proclaim liberty to captives" (Lk. 4:18). Jesus relentlessly reaches out to the people who are poor, hungry, sick, blind, deaf, leprous, paralyzed, or mentally ill. His care also includes sinners. This work, which the Creator gave Jesus to do (Jn. 17:4), shows the world God's redeeming love.

The following biblical references portray the compassion of Jesus. Moved with deep feelings at a leper's request of cure, Jesus ". . . stretched out his hand, touched him, and said: 'I do will it. Be cured'" (Mk. 1:41). This physical touch "cut through barriers of isolation and was a sign of Jesus' compassion and solidarity with suffering people."[10] Jesus entered the suffering of this leprous, social outcast living in misery. Jesus often touched the sick and disabled. Touch can speak more eloquently than words in time of grief or isolation.[11]

Jesus also taught what he modeled. The story of the Good Samaritan (Lk. 10:25-37) provides a powerful lesson about compassion toward those in need. Jesus verifies the law of love, ". . . love the Lord your God . . . and your neighbor as yourself" (v. 27-28), as living for eternal life. Next, Jesus answers the question, "Who is my neighbor?" (v. 29)

---

9. Patricia Normile, "Visiting the Sick: A Guide for Parish Ministers," *Church 8*, no. 2 (1992): 28-29.

10. Donald Senior, C.P., "Jesus the Physician: What the Gospels Say About Healing," in *Catholic Update*, ed. Jack Wintz, O.F.M. (Cincinnati: St. Anthony Messenger Press, 1990), 3.

11. Ibid.

by telling a story. A Samaritan, moved at the sight of the beaten and abandoned victim of robbery, cared for him (v. 30-35). The relationship of neighbor is determined by a person's attitude toward others, not by blood bonds, nationality, or religious community. By practicing love, the Samaritan – in contrast to the priest and Levite – shows he understood the law of love. He is neighbor to the robbed man.[12] Jesus refocuses the question. To act justly toward every person defines neighbor, not membership in a select group.[13] The lawyer concurs with Jesus: "the one who treated him with compassion" (v. 37) is neighbor, is loving. Jesus commands, "Do the same" (v. 37).

Further, Christian discipleship implies the care of the needy neighbor. Christians feed the hungry, give drink to the thirsty, offer hospitality to the homeless, clothe the naked, comfort the sick, and visit the imprisoned (Mt. 25:35-44). To act justly is to serve with compassion.

The Pastoral Care of the Sick: Rites of Anointing and Viaticum stresses the kind deeds required of the church toward those who are sick:

> The Church shows ... solicitude not only by visiting those who are in poor health but also by raising them up through the sacrament of anointing and by nourishing them with the Eucharist during their illness and when they are in danger of death. Finally, the Church offers prayers for the sick to commend them to God, especially in the last crisis of life (Decree).

In summary, sickness is a time of crisis. The sick need the help and support of others. It is a human ability to be compassionate. Compassion was the motivating force of Jesus' life. His human words and actions bespeak and confirm the tender and extravagant love of God. His compassionate transforming presence abides in and through his followers, the church (Mt. 16:18). With Jesus, they form one body (1 Cor. 12:12-27). For now, Christ's Body continues God's mission of compassionate love.

---

12. Jerome Kodell, O.S.B., "Luke," in *The Collegeville Bible Commentary*, eds. Dianne Bergant, C.S.A. and Robert J. Karris, O.F.M. (Collegeville: The Liturgical Press, 1989), 957.

13. Robert J. Karris, O.F.M., "The Gospel According to Luke," in *The New Jerome Biblical Commentary*, eds. Raymond E. Brown, S.S., Joseph A. Fitzmeyer, S.J. and Roland E. Murphy, O.Carm. (Englewood Cliffs: Prentice Hall, 1990), 702.

Objectives

The liturgical catechesis of this session will provide opportunity for the participants to achieve the following understanding and skills objectives:

Community

>by welcoming one another.

>by showing concern for those unable to participate in Sunday assembly.

Life

>by reflecting on personal experiences of sickness.

>by sharing experiences of sickness.

Faith

>by reflecting on the meaning of compassion in two biblical passages.

>by exploring how the church continues Christ's concern for the sick.

>by understanding the Eucharistic minister's healing presence to the sick.

Ministerial Skills

>by examining the church's rites for the sick and dying.

>by studying the introductory rite of *Communion of the Sick.*

Justice

>by affirming the rightful place of the sick in the Eucharistic community.

Ritual Prayer

>by praying together as community.

>by experiencing the supportive bond of communal prayer.

>by asking God for help in reaching out to the sick.

Preparation

Arrange the room in circular seating. Reserve a space within the room for ritual prayer. Create an ambience for prayer with an artistic arrangement of the Easter candle, table, cloth, opened Bible, glass bowl of water, leafy branch, and a living plant.

The day before the session, the persons proclaiming the word and those preparing refreshments are called to confirm their readiness. Calling the participants invites them anew. The materials needed are: Easter candle, table, cloth, Bible, glass bowl, water, leafy branch, living plant, song books, cassette player/tapes, *Communion of the Sick* for each participant, matches, catechist's notes, chart, handouts, movable chalk board/chalk/eraser, and refreshments.

The Catechetical Session

Welcome

The catechist greets each person by name and visits until it is time for the session. The catechist invites all to be seated.

Catechist: Welcome. Thank you for your bravery in risking new ministry. Look at all the support. (Gesture to group.) Let's introduce one another. Please partner with the person next to you. Learn about each other. Then, present one another to the group. (Introductions)

Gathering Prayer

Catechist: We have gathered. Shall we pray? (Pause) (Gesture with open hands and arms outstretched.) The Lord be with you.

All: And also with you.

Catechist: Let us pray.
God, Source of Love,
your redemptive presence is everlasting.
Help us to reach out to one another
with compassion and understanding.
We ask this in the name of Jesus,
through the power of the Holy Spirit.

All: Amen.

Life Experience

Catechist: The parish calls you to minister to the sick. Let us consider sickness which invades our lives. Each one has her or his story to share.
Here are some stories:
Entering her father's room, she heard him crying. "Dad, is the pain terrible?" "The pain is terrible; what is worse, this cancer claims my life." Clinging to his daughter, he cried, "I was angry and so afraid; you're here now; it's okay; we can talk and pray."(Pause)
Read story of women and visiting minister. (See catechist reflection).
Rain streaked down the window of Jane Lindstrom's hospital room. It deepened her feeling of loneliness and depression. Then someone brought a letter addressed to her. Jane opened it and read: "I missed your smile and your wave this morning, just as I have every morning since you've been ill. I pray you'll be well soon. You're probably surprised at receiving this note, but the world for me is a less happy place without you." Suddenly, Jane's feeling of loneliness and depression melted away. That brief note took a minute to write, but it was packed with love and power. It told Jane that she was missed and that she was remembered. "That knowledge," she said, "proved more effective than any medicine the doctor could prescribe."[14] (Pause)
Recall your experiences with sickness.
(Short Reflection)

Catechist: I invite you to share your experiences of sickness in small groups. Could you please move into groups of five? Would someone in the group jot down words or phrases to describe the effects of sickness?
(Small Group Discussion)

Catechist: To benefit from all your sharing, may we have two volunteers to list the effects of sickness on the chalk board as each recorder reports the group summary?
(Large Group Sharing)

---

14. Mark Link, S.J., "Sacrament of the Sick," in *The Catholic Vision* no. III-24 (Tabor Publishing, 1989), 1.

44 \ Eucharistic Ministry to the Sick

Possible Points for Sharing:
1. Sickness is a crisis of communication with oneself.
2. The stages of serious illness are periods of silence, aggression, depression, and acceptance.
3. Sickness is a crisis of communication with others.
4. Sickness is a crisis of communication with the church. (See Catechist Reflection.)

Catechist: In light of our discussion, how would we approach those who are sick as a healing presence? (Large Group Open Discussion)

Possible Points for Discussion:
1. The nature of compassion is "being one with." (See Catechist Reflection.)
2. These are some pastoral suggestions for visiting the sick.
    a) Have a sense of intentionality about what should happen during a visit to the sick.
    b) Conversation should center on the sick person.
    c) Accept the tension of sickness; do not try to force the atmosphere to be congenial.
    d) Comfort through facing, not avoiding, the situation.
    e) Help the person share thoughts and feelings.
    f) Be understanding and empathetic.
    g) Speak to what is, not to what should be.
    h) Be specific: what do you do, think, or feel?
    i) Be helpful by intimate sharing, not entertaining.
    j) Center conversation about people on significant relationships of the sick person.
    l) Nonverbal features of communication of presence are: open posture of uncrossed arms or legs, good eye contact, a feeling of relative relaxation, and responsive listening without fear of silence.[15]

---

15. Gusmer, 60-62.

Faith Reflection

Catechist: Jesus commands us to care for the sick. What meaning does Jesus attach to compassion in the gospel story of the Good Samaritan? How did Jesus show this compassion in touching a leper? (An Open Discussion.)

Possible Points for Discussion:

1. Concrete deeds of love are basic to Christian living.
2. How is neighbor defined?
3. Who is neighbor?
4. Physical touch cuts through barriers of isolation.
5. Touch speaks without words. (See Catechist Reflection.)

Catechist: From our shared experiences of human sickness, it is perceived as a disruption of normal life. Through the eyes of faith, what sense can be made of sickness and death? The *Pastoral Care of the Sick: Rites for Anointing and Viaticum* speaks to this in a section called "Human Sickness and Its Meaning in the Mystery of Salvation" (Gen Intro). Let us now consider this.
(See Appendix C for text of handouts.)
(An Open Discussion)

Catechist: The church continues Christ's concern for the sick. The church describes outreach to the sick in the *Pastoral Care of the Sick: Rites of Anointing and Viaticum*. Read the following:

> The rites in Part I . . . are used by the Church to comfort the sick in time of anxiety, to encourage them to fight against illness, and perhaps to restore them to health (Rite 42). The rites in Part II . . . are used by the Church to comfort and strengthen a Christian in the passage from this life. The ministry to the dying places emphasis on trust in the Lord's promise of eternal life . . . (Rite 161). Part I is entitled "Pastoral Care of the Sick," and Part II, "Pastoral Care of the Dying." Part I describes visits to the sick, communion to the sick, and the sacrament of anointing of the sick. Part II describes the celebration of viaticum, commendation of the dying, prayers for the dead, and rites for exceptional

circumstances. These are the specific liturgical rites the church offers for the care of the sick.

Who tends to this pastoral care? *The Introduction to the Rite* states:

> The concern that Christ showed for the bodily and spiritual welfare of those who are ill is continued by the Church in its ministry to the sick. This ministry is the common responsibility of all Christians, who should visit the sick, remember them in prayer, and celebrate the sacraments with them. The family and friends of the sick, doctors and others who care for them, and priests with pastoral responsibilities have a particular share in this ministry of comfort. Through words of encouragement and faith they can help the sick to unite themselves with the sufferings of Christ for the good of God's people (Rite 43).

Lay ministers may preside at the visiting and communion rites of the sick. The priest is the usual presider at the rite of anointing and the rites of the dying. As Eucharistic ministers, why are you a healing presence to the sick? A three-fold answer is expressed in *Ministers of Care:*

> As a representative from your faith commuity, you are to be yourself, but to be from others. You come to a particular person in faith to witness . . . faith is alive in your local community, these Christians truly do love one another.
>
> Second, you are to engage this person in a relationship, (one that helps the person) come to know Jesus through faith. . . . You need to give life and to encourage and develop the kind of relationship that allows people to trust themselves, to trust you, to trust the Lord.
>
> Third, you are a prayerful example of God's presence. You are also a witness of your own personal faith: This is what God's presence in my life means to me.[16]

---

16. Marilyn Kofler and Kevin O'Connor, *Handbook for Ministers of Care* (Chicago: Liturgical Training Publication, 1987), 6-7.

Now, let us enjoy the refreshments prepared for us by (Names). After break, we will gather in the prayer space. (Break)

Ritual Prayer

(Catechist invites everyone to gather for prayer.)

Call to Prayer

Catechist: God so wonderfully loves us at all times. With grateful hearts for all God's gifts, let us sing our thanks and praise.

Gathering Song

"God of Day and God of Darkness"[17]

Scriptural Reading

(Catechist lights the Easter candle.)

Narrator: A reading from the Gospel of Luke.

All: Praise to you Lord, Jesus Christ.

Narrator: On one occasion a lawyer stood up to pose him this problem:

Lawyer: Teacher, what must I do to inherit everlasting life?

Jesus: What is written in the law? How do you read it?

Lawyer: You shall love the Lord your God with all your heart, with all your soul, with all your strength, and with all your mind; and your neighbor as yourself.

Jesus: You have answered correctly. Do this and you shall live.

Narrator: Wishing to justify himself, he asked:

Lawyer: And who is my neighbor?

Jesus: A man going down from Jerusalem to Jericho fell prey to robbers. They stripped and beat him, leaving him half-dead. A priest, going down the same road, saw him but continued on. A Levite who came the same way saw him and went on. A Samaritan journeying along came on him and he was

---

17. Robert J. Batastini, General Editor, *Gather* (Chicago: GIA Publications, Inc., 1988), 319. (v. 1-3)

48 \ *Eucharistic Ministry to the Sick*

> moved to pity at the sight. He approached him, and dressed his wounds, pouring in oil and wine. He then hoisted him on his own beast and brought him to an inn, where he cared for him. The next day he gave the innkeeper two silver pieces with the request: look after him. I will pay any further expense on my way back. Which of these three, in your opinion, was neighbor to the man who fell in with robbers?

Lawyer: The one who treated him with compassion.

Jesus: Then go and do the same.

Narrator: The Gospel of the Lord.

All: Praise to you, Lord Jesus Christ.

Response to the Word

(Moment of Silence) (Catechist gestures all to be seated.)

Reflection Tape: "St. Teresa's Prayer" John Michael Talbot.[18]

Receiving the Book Containing the Rite of Communion of the Sick

(Catechist stands and gestures for all to stand.)

Catechist: (Name), receive *The Rite of Communion of the Sick.* May you bear Christ to the sick. (The catechist calls each person by name.)

Petitions

Catechist: In our joy and sorrow, we come before the Lord. In prayer, let us present our needs. (Pause) For ministers in the Church, we pray . . .

All: Lord, hear our prayer.

Catechist: For the sick, especially for (Names of Parish Sick), we pray . . .
For peace among nations, we pray . . .
For what else shall we pray?

Catechist: Gathering our prayers and praises into one,
we pray as Jesus taught us:

---

18. *Quiet Reflections,* produced and directed by Billy Ray Hearn and Phil Perkins (Canoga Park: The Sparrow Corporation, 1987), audiocassette.

All: Our Father . . .

Closing Prayer

Catechist: Gentle God, you are our source of strength.
Let not fear keep us from finding you in others,
especially the sick.
This we ask in the name of Jesus,
through the power of the Holy Spirit.

All: Amen.

Closing Song

"God of Day and God of Darkness"[19]

Skills of Ministry

Catechist: Take a few minutes to look at your copy of *Communion of the Sick*. Let us again situate this rite in the whole outreach of the church to the sick. You have Chapter III of *The Pastoral Care of the Sick*. On page three in the Contents, you notice a rite for *Communion in Ordinary Circumstances* and one for *Communion in a Hospital or Institution*. The one we will study and usually use is *Communion in Ordinary Circumstances*.

(Use a chart to explain the composition of the rite; see Appendix D for an outline.)

The format appears similar to the celebration of Eucharist. The rite provides for communion to the sick in context of a liturgy of the word. We want to look specifically at the introductory rite. It consists of three parts: greeting, sprinkling rite, and penitential rite. The purpose of introductory rites is to render a sense of coming together before the Lord.

The greeting brings to focus that we are in the presence of the Lord. As an expression of wish, not statement, the greeting keeps a sense of prayer. "The Lord be with you" is a prayer of the presider that the sick and those gathered are indeed experiencing being present together before the Lord.[20]

---

19. Gather, 319, (vs. 4-5).
20. Ralph Keifer, *To Give Thanks and Praise* (Washington, D.C.: The Pastoral Press, 1986), 109.

The representative from the parish celebration of Eucharist unites the sick to the worshipping community from which they are separated.

The sprinkling rite, as #82 suggests, "calls to mind our baptism into Christ." In the baptismal waters, Christians are "plunged into the Paschal Mystery of Christ" (CLS 6). We are initiated into Christ, into his dying and rising, into the faith community. Look at the instructions #82. You will find this part is designated for the priest or deacon. The word "minister" indicates you as a presider. You may preside at the rite of sprinkling of the sick. The pastor decided this because similiar rites authorize "the minister" to preside at the sprinkling rite.[21]

The wording of the penitential rite makes this appear to be a time to examine our consciences. However, more appropriately, it calls people to a remembrance of God's mercy. The "Lord Have Mercy" is a litany. A litany expresses, by its rhythmic repetition, a sense of being present to the Lord. It is an expressive statement of love, honor, and devotion.[22] Look at the organization of the texts. There are a number of options given. Keeping in mind the sick to whom you are taking communion, choose the prayer that is most appropriate. Preparing for ministry in liturgy ensures a more focused and prayerful celebration. We have considered the meaning of the Introductory Rite in light of faith. Now, let us actually practice being presider at this prayer. Break into your small groups. One person can take the role of presider and the others the assembly. Then, switch roles.

(Role Play)

Just Service

Catechist: In this session, we have focused on sickness, outreach to the sick, the church's concern, and the Eucharistic minister's healing presence to the sick. The perspective used was that of our response to those who are sick, more specifically, to those

---

21. National Conference of Catholic Bishops, *Catholic Household Blessings & Prayers* (Washington, D.C.: United States Catholic Conference, 1988), 257.
22. Keifer, 112-113.

unable to be at the Eucharistic table, including those suffering with AIDS. Let us view this action in a larger context. Vatican II tells us "the Church has a single intention: that God's kingdom may come."[23] God's Kingdom

> is God insofar as God is redemptively present and active in the human heart, in the midst of a group of people, in a community, in institutions and movements, in the world at large, in nature, in the cosmos. The Kingdom of God exists whenever and wherever the will of God is acknowledged and fulfilled.[24]

Jesus is the redemptive presence of God. For now, Jesus acts through the church. Jesus defined human ministry for the sake of the realm of God. In Matthew 25:31-46, Jesus equates Christian discipleship with care for those in need.[25] Christians feed the hungry, offer hospitality to the homeless, give drink to the the thirsty, clothe the naked, comfort the sick, and visit the imprisoned. This service is a matter of acting justly (Micah 6:8).

Therefore, for us to participate in the Church's care of the sick is to perform a work of mercy. In doing works of mercy, we are the redemptive presence of God. We are active in bringing about God's realm.

Preparation for Next Session

I invite you to prepare for participation in the next session on the liturgy of the word. Prayerfully study a reading from #84 (pgs. 14-16) or one from Part III of *Communion of the Sick* beginning on page 30. You may share your reflections in small group.

---

23. Vatican II, "Pastoral Constitution on the Chruch in the Modern World," in *Vatican Council II: The Conciliar and Post Conciliar Documents,* Vol. 1, ed. Austin Flannery, O.P. (Northport: Costello Publishing Company, 1988), 45.

24. Richard McBrien, *Ministry* (San Francisco: Harper and Row, 1987), 22.

25. Benedict T. Viviano, O.P., "The Gospel According to Matthew," in *New Jerome Biblical Commentary,* eds. Raymond E. Brown, S.S., Joseph Fitzmyer, S.J. and Roland E. Murphy, O.Carm. (Englewood Cliffs: Prentice Hall, 1990), 669.

Dismissal Prayer

Sprinkling Rite

(Catechist lifts the bowl of water.)

Catechist: We were baptized into Christ who by his death and resurrection has redeemed us (Adapted from Rite 82).

Song

(With leafy branch, catechist sprinkles all during song.)
"Water of Life"[26]

Blessing

(All extend hands in blessing.)

Catechist: May God bless us and keep us. May God be gracious to us and give us peace in the name of Jesus, through the power of the Holy Spirit (Adapted from Rite 91).

All: Amen.

(The session ends. The catechist thanks all for coming and for their participation. The catechist bids them farewell.)

Session Two:
The Community Listens and Responds in Faith

Catechist Reflection

Stories capture the happenings of life. The life and faith stories of individuals are unique, yet general. Every human life has the common relationships of self, family and friends, society and institution, universe and God. No individual has been, is, or will be exactly like another. However, elements in each person's life and faith story transcend the particular details and apply to everyone.[27]

Storytelling is inherent to human living. Human lives create the story content. Sharing stories enable their continuance. Further, reflected story makes possible its influence on the teller and listeners alike. Cir-

---

26. David Haas, *Who Calls You by Name* (Chicago: GIA Publications, Inc., 1988), 47.
27. John Shea, *Stories of God* (Chicago: The Thomas More Press, 1978), 11-39.

cumstances of life can shape the story of individuals. Yet, the story of individuals can shape these circumstances, can touch the lives of other people.

In a larger sense, our stories are part of God's story. Our lives are intertwined with the story of who God is. In the telling of God's story, we realize who we are. Stories of God set out God's relationship with us and our possible relationship with God. John Shea states: "The stories of God are not solely about God or about us but the terrifying distance and incredible closeness between us."[28]

Storytelling was the original vehicle for passing on the people's faith in God and identity with God. Carol Luebering explains:

> When words strike home in the hearts of believers, people who are consciously searching for an understanding of the God who dwells with them and within them, they recognize God's voice in the words. And when such people remember a story or insight and pass it down from generation to generation, when folks far down the line still find that it resonates with their experience of life and of God, then the community of believers begins to insist that something in those words, time-bound though they are, holds timeless truth. . . . That's how we got . . . the writings we call Scripture.[29]

Scripture is rich in its many stories of God. The creation story and the covenant between God and the Israelites demonstrate the love of God. Jesus fulfills the telling of God's story of love for humanity. The story of Jesus began in the "mysterious design which for all ages was hidden in God" (Eph. 3:9). Jesus revealed God's act of redemption "by the total fact of his presence and self-manifestation – by words and works, signs and miracles, but above all by his death and resurrection from the dead, and finally, by sending the Spirit of Truth."[30] This salvific mission of Jesus is told in the gospel stories.

Within these stories, Jesus defines his own image as a "physician." Once, when his opponents attack him for having among his disciples unsavory characters such as tax collectors and sinners, Jesus reminds them that "those who are well do not need a physician, but the sick do"

---

28. Ibid., 64.

29. Carol Luebering, *Ministers of the Lord's Presence: Lectors' Edition* (Cincinnati: St. Anthony Messenger Press, 1990), 26-27.

30. Vatican II, "Dogmatic Constitution on Divine Revelation," in *Vatican Council II: The Conciliar and Post Conciliar Documents*, Vol. 1, ed. Austin Flannery, O.P. (Northport: Costello Publishing Company, 1988), 4.

(Mk. 2:17). In his initial preaching in his hometown synagogue of Nazareth, Jesus challenges the congregation: "Surely you will quote me this proverb, 'Physician, cure yourself,' and say, 'Do here in your native place the things that we heard were done in Capernaum'" (Lk. 4:23). The crowds seem instinctively to see Jesus as "physician." "They brought him those who were ill and possessed by demons" (Mk. 2:32). Further,

> . . . his reputation traveled the length of Syria. They carried to him all those afflicted with various diseases and racked with pain: the possessed, the lunatics, the paralyzed. He cured them all (Mt. 4:24).

The Gospels note the remarkable attention Jesus gives to the sick. Much of his time is consumed with encounters with people who are sick, blind, lame, deaf, leprous, paralyzed, or mentally ill.

As Jesus went about his healing ministry, touch was a very important activity for him. Turning to a healing story in the Gospel of Mark (1:40-45), we find one example of the role of touch in Jesus ministry of healing:

> A leper approached Jesus with a request, kneeling down as he addressed him: "If you will to do so, you can cure me." Moved with pity, Jesus stretched out his hand, touched him, and said: "I will do it. Be cured." The leprosy left him then and there, and he was cured. Jesus gave him a stern warning and sent him on his way. "Not a word to anyone, now," he said. "Go off and present yourself to the priest and offer for your cure what Moses prescribed. That should be proof for them." The man went off and began to proclaim the whole matter freely, making the story public. As a result of this, it was no longer possible for Jesus to enter a town openly. He stayed in desert places, yet people kept coming to him from all sides.

The passage reveals that Jesus was not afraid to touch those who were feared and despised by his society. In many ways, people with HIV and AIDS are treated as modern day lepers. Fear and disapproval keep many people at a distance. But people with HIV and AIDS need the healing touch of compassion as much as any sick person does.

As you prepare to hear the stories of people with HIV and AIDS as part of your ministry to the sick, it is good to reflect on the importance of touch in the ministry of healing, and to examine your own feelings about touching a person with HIV or AIDS. If fear is present, it would be good to surface that fear, examine it, and find ways to overcome it, before visiting a person with HIV or AIDS.

The Good News of the Gospels is that this man Jesus is the real presence of God among us. The men and women of the time of Jesus remembered and embodied the words, actions, and teachings of Jesus. Through the Spirit, Jesus continues to be present to the community of believers. The Gospels enable christian disciples today to believe that Jesus is Messiah, the Son of God. They challenge christian communities to live the christian way set forth by Jesus.

It is through the medium of story that the minister of care relates to the sick. He or she compassionately listens to their stories: the stories of isolation caused by suffering and loneliness, of anger and fear, of depression, and of acceptance of illness. By sharing the gospel story of Jesus with the sick, the minister helps them make connections between their story and the story of God. Their story is part of God's relationship with them. The sick are invited beyond their human pain to the hope their faith offers in the acceptance of God in their lives. The church's liturgy for the sick, *Communion of the Sick,* calls them into an experience of the presence of God. The minister of care presides at this liturgy of proclaiming the Word and sharing the Bread.

In summary, story is the narrative of life. The common ground of humanity allows any human story to touch others and even challenge them. The stories of God inevitably include humanity. The gospel stories of Jesus invite us to believe in God's love and compassion; they challenge our way of thinking and acting. The teachings and actions of Jesus are continued in and through the Church. The ministers of the sick use the medium of story, both human and divine, to relate to the sick. Through liturgy, the sick experience the presence of God in the proclamation of the Word and the sharing of the Bread.

Objectives

The liturgical catechesis of this session will provide an opportunity for the participants to achieve these objectives in the experience of:

Community

    by greeting one another.

    by participating in a communal action of faith, the proclamation of the word.

Life

    by reflecting on human life through story.

by sharing the experience of listening to another's story.

Faith

by reflecting on a biblical story's connection to the human story of sickness and pain.

by understanding the proclamation of the word in the light of faith.

Ministerial Skills

by studying the liturgy of the word of *The Rite of Communion of the Sick.*

by reviewing pastoral aspects of proclaiming the Word.

Justice

by realizing the right of the sick to receive communion in context of the Liturgy of the Word.

Ritual Prayer

by praying together as community.

by experiencing the supportive bond of communal prayer.

by giving thanks, worshipping God.

Preparation

Arrange the room in circular seating. Reserve a space within the room for ritual prayer. Create an ambience for prayer with an artistic arrangement of the Easter candle, table, cloth, opened Bible, incense, clay pot, charcoal, and a living plant.

The day before the session, the person proclaiming the word and those preparing refreshments are called to confirm their readiness. The materials needed are: Easter candle, table, cloth, Bible, incense, clay pot, charcoal, matches, cassette player/tapes, movable chalk board/chalk/eraser, overhead projector/transparencies, song books, catechist's notes, handouts, living plant, and refreshments.

The Catechetical Session

Welcome

The participants and catechist greet one another by name and visit until it is time for the session. The catechist invites all to be seated.

Gathering Prayer

Catechist: It is good to see each of you again. Let us continue our gathering in prayer. (Pause) (Gesture with open hands and arms outstretched.) The Lord be with you.

All: And also with you.

Catechist: God, Teller of salvation story,
You told your story through the Word made flesh.
Inspire us to accept the invitation of challenge
that the life of Jesus offers.
We ask this in his name,
through the power of his Spirit.

All: Amen.

Life Experience

Catechist: "Letter from Jim,"[31] a story from Garrison Keillor's public radio show featuring "News from Lake Wobegon," depicts events of an individual within that community. Are you able to identify with aspects of the storyteller's account? Do these life experiences resonate with your or others' life experiences? Listen and find out. (Listening To Story)

Catechist: What did you learn about the community of Lake Wobegon? (Discuss; then, ask next question.) What are some of the common aspects of life in the story with which you can identify? Who/what influenced Jim's decision? Why had Jim come to this point in his life? What happened as a result of this decision? How did it affect the community? Why is

---

31. Garrison Keillor, *News from Lake Wobegon: Spring,* produced and directed by Lynne Cruise, Margaret Moos and Tom Mudge, 11.52 min. (Lake Wobegon: Minnesota Public Radio, 1983), audiocassette.

Garrison a good story teller? What made you a good listener? What have you learned about the medium of story?

Possible Points for Discussion:

1. The content of story consists of the happenings of everyday life.
2. The retelling and listening enables the continuance of the individual's story, which can apply to everyone.
3. Reflected story makes possible its influence on the teller and listeners. (See Catechist Reflection.)

Faith Reflection

Catechist: Your ministry to the sick involves the medium of story. You listen to the stories of the sick, such as we discussed last session: stories of isolation, of anger and fear, of depression and of acceptance of illness. You listen with full attention and compassion. You ask questions to elicit the thinking and feelings of the sick. Sometimes we tell them stories. We tell them the Jesus story which we call the Proclamation of the Word. This is similar to what we do on Sunday. As ministers to the sick, we continuously make connections between the story of the Jesus and the story of the sick. We enable the sick persons to recognize their story as part of the Jesus story, as part of God's relationship with them.

Do you recall our discussion of the meaning of human sickness in the mystery of salvation? Through faith, sickness and suffering has meaning and value for our own salvation and for the salvation of the world. The human story becomes part of the divine story. In Christ, human pain and suffering become redemptive. The sick are healed in spirit. To be healed in this way does not mean that the pain or sufferings will be taken away. Rather, it means their pain becomes part of a greater pain and their experience part of the greater experience of Christ. Stories of Jesus' suffering told and listened to in faith assist us in this truth.

Let us reflect on a suggested text of the rite for the Proclamation of the Word and relate it to the story of the sick. Jesus says: "I am the true vine, you are the branches. He who lives in me and I in him, will produce abundantly, for apart from me you can do nothing (Jn. 15:5).

A Catechetical Process for Preparing Ministers to the Sick / 59

(Open Discussion)

Possible Points for Discussion:

1. The vine and its branches are most closely connected. The vine is the source of life, nourishment, and support to the branches.
2. Baptism grafts us into Jesus Christ. Through the sacramental life of the church, we continue to draw life from the life of Christ.
3. In weakness and sickness, we draw strength by the mystery of participating in God's life. The church's eucharistic celebration nourishes and strengthens our union with Jesus Christ through the proclaiming the Word and the sharing of the Bread.
4. We believe we live in Jesus and Jesus lives in us, helping us to produce good fruit: love for the sick, patience in our pain and suffering, repentance, thankfulness, peace of mind and soul.

Catechist: In light of our faith, we gather to listen to the Word of God being proclaimed. What do we believe about this action of faith?

(Ask a participant to read aloud CSL 7.)

> ... Christ is always present in his Church, especially in its liturgical celebrations. He is present in the sacrifice of the Mass, not only in the person of his minister, . . . but especially under the Eucharistic elements. . . . He is present in his word, since it is he himself who speaks when the holy Scriptures are read in the Church. He is present, lastly, when the Church prays and sings, for he promised: "Where two or three are gathered together in my name, there am I in the midst of them" (Mt. 18:20) (CSL 7). (See Handout from the above selection for each participant.)

(Using a transparency with only the important phrases, have the participants underline these special ways Christ is present; see Appendix E for this transparency.)

(Open Discussion)

Possible Points for Discussion:

1. The Christian community believes Sacred Scripture is inspired revelation. In communal listening to the proclamation of the Word,

members of the celebrating community – in this case, those who are sick – believe God is present.[32]

2. Christ's presence in the Word makes the Word nourishment for Christians. In Christ's presence the celebrating community continues to be nourished.[33]

Catechist: The liturgy of the sick is a celebration of the presence of Christ. The liturgy of the Word not only informs people of a message from God, but brings them into communion with the God of the message. I invite you to share your reflections on the Scripture text you had chosen with your small group. Please move into groups of five.
(Small Group Sharing)
Enjoy the refreshments prepared for us by (Names).

Skills of Ministry

Catechist: The Liturgy of the Word consists of the proclamation of Scripture, the response and general petitions. We believe that God is present in the midst of God's people in the proclaiming of the Word. How can Liturgy of the Word say: "I am your God, you are my people, close to my heart?" What facets of the celebration of the Word signal this presence?
We proclaim the Word from the Lectionary, Bible, or book meant for proclamation. *The General Introduction to the Lectionary for Mass* states:

> The books containing the readings of the Word of God remind the hearers of the presence of God speaking to his (sic) people. Since, in liturgical celebrations the books serve as signs and symbols of the sacred, . . . ensure . . . they are truly worthy and beautiful (LMI 35). Because of the dignity of the Word of God, the books of reading used in the celebration are not to be replaced by other pastoral aids. . . . (LMI 37)[34]

---

32. Robert D. Duggan, "Sunday Eucharist: Theological Reflections," *Chicago Studies* 29, no. 3 (1990), 217-219.

33. Kevin W. Irwin, Liturgy, *Prayer and Spirituality* (Ramsey: Paulist Press, 1984), 99-100.

34. *Sa*cred Congregation for the Sacraments and Divine Worship, "General Introduction to the Lectionary for Mass," in *Vatican Council II: More Post Conciliar Documents*, Vol. 2, ed. Austin Flannery, O.P. (Collegeville: The Liturgical Press, 1982). Hereafter referred to as LMI with paragraph number.

What does this say to a lector or to you in your ministry to the sick? (Accept comments.)

What does this say to a lector or to you in your ministry to the sick? (Accept comments.)

Who proclaims the word when you preside at the liturgy of the sick? Rite #84 states: it "is proclaimed by one of those present or by the minister." That more people might share their gifts in the celebration, it would be best if someone other than the presider proclaim the Word if possible.

What is required of the usual lector or of ourselves in proclaiming the Word? Ralph Keifer targets this requirement for proclamation:

> Most simply and critically put, the bread of God's Word must be broken in faith by the faithful ministers. But because liturgy is a proclamation intended to express faith openly, it is not enough that readers and homilists believe in their heart of hearts. Their faith must also be perceptible in what they do and say as they perform the ministry of the Word. This requires training, study, and preparation.[35]

What does this say to you as minister to the sick? (Accept comments.)

The directives for Response to the Word include a period of silence (#85). What is the significance of this silence? It plays an important part in sustaining the atmosphere of prayer and praise. Measured pause, or silence, allows time to relate the human story to the Word, to prepare response to it in prayer and to enable the work of the Spirit (LMI 28).

The "brief explanation of the reading" called for by the rite can take many forms (#85). If you take communion to the sick from the Sunday assembly and use the Sunday readings, you might like to summarize the presider's homily. Quoting Father (Name) may bring further realization that this rite of communion flows from the eucharistic celebration of the parish. You could offer a few words of your own reflections applying it to the needs of the sick. You may have a shared reflection with those present or with the sick person. Short

---

35. Keifer, 122.

commentaries on some of the scripture readings on pages 34-38 of *Communion of the Sick* will assist you.

Why is it important to proclaim the Word and reflect on the Word when we visit the sick? In the Eucharistic celebration, the faithful are invited to the table of the Word and Sacrament. The Word helps us to understand Eucharist and leads into its celebration. Christ is present in the proclamation of the Word; to break open the Word is "to release the God who lives there."[36] Listening to the word and sharing the Bread are nourishment to the faith of the sick.

We respond to God's Word in petitions called General Intercessions. We ask God to help the sick live out the Word and deal with problems and needs the sick have at the moment. In celebrating the Liturgy of the Word with the sick, it is well to remember that sickness tends to narrow one's vision of the world. You might prepare intentions related to world, country, parish. This helps those who are sick reconnect with the larger community. Invite intentions of prayer from the sick person and those present. You will find selections of general intercessions to refer to for use as guides on pages 39-43 of *Communion of the Sick*.

Let us break into our small groups and practice proclaiming the Word. You might want to proclaim the text you prepared for this class.
(Role Play)

Just Service

Catechist: In this session, we have considered the dynamics within any human story to challenge the lives of others. We recalled how the stories of God involve us. The Gospel stories of Jesus invite us to believe in God's love and compassion, especially for the sick. Jesus challenges our way of thinking and acting. The stories of Jesus are remembered in and through the Church. This happens in proclaiming the Word of Scripture and celebrating Eucharist. We focused on proclaiming the Word, especially to the sick.

---

36. Shea, 73.

The Liturgy of the Word is part of *Communion of the Sick in Ordinary Circumstances*. The Church has given this rite in behalf of "the faithful who are ill" and "deprived of their rightful and accustomed place in the Eucharistic community" (Rite 73). The *Commentary* of the rite voices the desire of the Church. "When at all possible, the full rite with the liturgy of the word is to be preferred"[37] to the rite for use in the hospital. This makes it very clear that in ordinary circumstances, the full rite should be used. The table of the Word is the rightful nourishment of the sick. It is the responsibility of the minister to prepare and preside at the full rite to assure the sick this opportunity of participating in the sharing of Word, as well as sharing in the Bread.

Preparation for Next Session

I invite you to prepare for participation in the next session, liturgy of holy communion. Please watch the film *Places in the Heart* and reflect on the human community. Here are three copies of the film. How would you like to handle the viewing? I am willing to set up the VCR here a number of times this week or you could watch with a group at someone's home, or pass the films around. (Decision) Please take a copy of questions for reflection on the film. (See Appendix F for the questions to be copied.)

Ritual Prayer

(Catechist invites everyone to move to the prayer space and presents psalm copies to them.)

Call to Prayer

Catechist: God has spoken love and mercy through Jesus.
　　　　　For the gift of Jesus
　　　　　let us sing our thanks and praise.

---

37. Commentary: *Pastoral Care of the Sick*, 5.

64 \ *Eucharistic Ministry to the Sick*

Gathering Song

"We Have Been Told"[38]

Psalmody

    All: If today you hear God's voice, harden not your hearts.

Side One: O Come, let us sing to our God; let us make a joyful noise to the rock of our salvation.

Side Two: We come into your presence with thanksgiving, rejoicing with songs of praise. For you, God, are our God, a great Ruler over all other gods.

Side One: We bow down before you and worship, kneeling before you, our Maker. For you are our God, and we are your people, the flock that you shepherd.

Side Two: Today let us hearken to your voice: "Harden not your hearts, as at Meribah, as on the day at Massah in the desert, when your ancestors tested me, and put me to the test, though they had seen my works" (Ps 95).

Side One: Glory to you, Source of all Being, Eternal Word, and Holy Spirit

Side Two: As it was in the beginning, is now, and will be forever. Amen.

    All: If today you hear God's voice, harden not your hearts.

Gospel Acclamation

(Catechist lights the Easter candle. After putting incense on the lighted charcoal, she or he reverently incenses the Bible and the group during the Gospel acclamation.)

    "Word of Truth and Life"[39] (Sing along with refrain on tape.)

Scriptural Reading

Lector: A reading from the Gospel of Luke.

    All: Praise to you Lord, Jesus Christ.

Lector: Jesus came to Nazareth where he had been reared. Entering the synagogue on the sabbath as he was in the habit of doing,

---

38. Gather, 296. (v. 1-2)

39. Marty Haugen, *Mass of Creation* (Chicago: GIA Publications, Inc., 1985), audiocassette.

he stood up to do the reading. When handed a scroll of the prophet Isaiah, he unrolled the scroll and found the passage where it was written: "The Spirit of the Lord is upon me, because he has anointed me to bring glad tidings to the poor. He has sent me to proclaim liberty to captives and recovery of sight to the blind, to let the oppressed go free, and to proclaim a year acceptable to the Lord." Rolling up the scroll, he handed it back to the attendant and sat down. The eyes of all in the synagogue looked intently at him. He said to them, "Today this Scripture passage is fulfilled in your hearing." All . . . were amazed at the gracious words that came from his mouth.
The Gospel of the Lord.

All: Praise to you, Lord Jesus Christ.

Response to the Word

(Moment of Silence) (Catechist gestures all to be seated.)

Catechist: Let us share our reflections on the message of the Word, or about the God who spoke it. (Pause) When the story resonates with the familiar, with the experience of our life, the story awakens us, draws us in. This happened to Jesus in this scripture text. In the midst of the gathered community, Jesus is lector. His faith is perceptible in proclaiming the words of the prophet Isaiah. As part of the gathered people, he too ponders the word. Jesus had experienced the "Spirit of the Lord" at his baptism and during his time in the desert. He could enter the story and identify with the prophet from of old.

The work of the prophet was now his mission. He would bear out the words of Scripture in his living. Jesus would respond by reaching out to those who were economically, physically, and socially marginalized. Jesus saw himself as good news to the poor. Jesus is the presence of a God of love and compassion. (Pause) Please feel free to share your reflections.

(Reflection)

66 \ *Eucharistic Ministry to the Sick*

Petitions

Catechist: We stand before God whose presence sustains us.
In prayer, let us present our needs. (Pause)
For renewed faith, we pray . . .

All: Lord, hear our prayer.

Catechist: For the marginated people of our society, we pray . . .
For the sick, especially for (Names of Parish Sick), we pray . . .
For what else shall we pray?

Catechist: For these needs and those unspoken, we pray as Jesus taught us:

All: Our Father . . .

Closing Prayer

Catechist: God, Faithful Presence, we have listened to your word and shared reflections on its meaning. May we cherish your word in our hearts, share it with our brothers and sisters, and live it out in our lives. We pray in the name of Jesus through the power of the Holy Spirit.

All: Amen.

Closing Song

"We Have Been Told"[40]

(The session ends. The catechist thanks all for coming and for their participation. The catechist bids them farewell.)

Session Three:
The Community Unites in Celebrative Sharing

Catechist Reflection

In the "Family Matters" section of *Living Waters,* the family is perceived as a unit of belonging where we live out our most imtimate and powerful human experiences. The family is connected with ties that

---

40. Gather, 296. (v. 2-3)

bind. These ties are trust, sacrifice, and care. Trust allows individual family members to be creative and to take risks that enable growth. Sacrifice enhances the bond of unity by maintaining the perspective of family. This means living a simple life style, living in ways that support family. Care reflects the giving and the receiving inherent in a family. These ties of trust, sacrifice, and care bind individuals into a compassionate family. Family, then, "is where you can be underfoot and understood all at the same time."[41]

Of all the things a family does, eating together is the most important. In sharing a meal, family members do more than share food and drink. They share who they are for one another. The food and drink they share become tokens of their flesh and blood. The individual members become food and drink for one another: nourishment, sustenance, and support for one another. The family meal celebrates the loving bonds that grow in family whenever the members set about the business of being family, the daily tasks involved in the living of family.[42]

Family, then, can be a place where one finds love, understanding, and support, even when all else fails. Here, one can be refreshed and recharged to cope more effectively with the world outside. Yet, not to measure up, to fall short of the ideal relationship, is part of being human also. Reconciling love bridges chasms of fear, dishonesty and hatred. Reconciliation enables freedom to be true to self, a reuniting or building of a relationship, a deeper growth into community.

The film *Places in the Heart*[43] portrays a time, a place, and a people – a community. The story enters the lives of specific families torn, reborn, and bonded in ways other than blood. *Places in the Heart* is a story of human courage and tenderness. It is equally a story of human sinfulness, of prejudice, hatred, and adultery. The drama begins with a scene in the distance of people coming from the church with the background music of "Blessed Assurance." You meet the characters by quick flashes of each family at a meal. At the end of the film, the members of the congregation pass the communion plate from hand to hand, wishing one another "peace of God." We see the whole human church: rich and poor, black and white, the loving and the unloving, the oppressor and the victim, the strong and the weak, the living and the dead.

---

41. Anne Marie Mongoven, O.P., Ph.D., and Maureen Gallagher, Ph.D., *Living Waters*, Text 2 (Allen, TX: Tabor Publishing, 1991), 4.

42. Ibid., 118.

43. Robert Benton, *Places in the Heart*, produced and directed by Arlene Donovan and Robert Benton, 113 min., CBS/Fox Video, 1984, videocassette.

Out of such diversity, the Lord calls us to community. If we look to ourselves or back in history, Christians have had difficulty getting along with each other. Nevertheless, our faith insists that community is possible. Believing ears still hear Jesus' Last Supper command: "This is how all know you for my disciples: your love for one another" (Jn. 13:35). The *Didache,* one of the oldest Eucharistic prayers in our Christian tradition, prays for unity born from diversity like grains of wheat ground into flour:

> Just as the bread broken
> was first scattered on the hills,
> then gathered and became one,
> so let your Church be gathered . . . .[44]

At the meal of Eucharist, the prayers remind us we are gathered in God's presence, who God is, and what God dreams for us. We hear the story of what God has done for us in Jesus. We share the nourishment which makes us his Body. We are one with Christ and with one another. The presence of Jesus transforms us into a community, his living Body on earth.

"That they might be one" (Jn. 17:11) was the prayer and effort of Jesus' entire life, death, and resurrection. He liberated the sinners and reached out in service to the poor, the sick, the widow, and the orphan. By washing the feet of his disciples at the Last Supper (Jn. 13:1-17), Jesus symbolically shows what Eucharist is about; it connects Eucharist with service. Jesus gave them a mission of service: "As I have done, so you must do" (v. 15); love "as I have loved you" (Jn. 15:12). The tools Jesus left his disciples were a basin and towel. These are the tools of a servant. It was the work of a servant he wished them to do. The towel and basin makes demands on us as Christians. We are commissioned to make contact with those who are considered to be among the "less attractive" members of humanity, and carry out our ministry with loving attention. We must transcend our own self interest to minister to the sick, the poor, and needy in their pain and suffering.[45]

As your ministry brings us into contact with persons with HIV and AIDS, you have the opportunity to extend a welcome to them as members of the great, diverse human family, the Christian community.

---

44. *Didache,* 9-10.

45. R. Kevin Seasoltz, "Justice and Eucharist," in *Living Bread,* Saving Cup, ed. R. Kevin Seasoltz (Collegeville: The Liturgical Press, 1987), 316-320.

A Catechetical Process for Preparing Ministers to the Sick / 69

The Christian community Jesus envisioned is larger than any small gathering, larger even than the Sunday assembly. It is what *Places in the Heart* showed us on a small scale. It is a gathering of saints and sinners, the living and the dead. The Christian community is a people who have shared bread, who reach out to embrace the stranger, even the unlovable. They continue to gather in the Lord's name and in the Lord's presence to be nourished, to be made one. They remember the sick members unable to gather; they take the nourishment of Eucharist to these sick members.

Objectives

The liturgical catechesis of this session will provide opportunity for the participants to achieve these objectives in the experience of:

Community

by welcoming one another.
by preparing to take communion to those unable to participate in the Sunday assembly.

Life

by reflecting on the interaction of a human community through a film.
by sharing the experience of the community in the film.

Faith

by exploring the meaning of Eucharist in John 13: 1-17.
by relating Eucharist as service to the ministry of taking communion to the sick.

Ministerial Skills

by studying the liturgy of holy communion of *The Rite of Communion of the Sick*.
by reviewing pastoral aspects of giving communion to the sick.

Justice

by actualizing the right of the sick to receive communion.

Ritual Prayer

> by praying together as community.
> by experiencing the supportive bond of communal prayer.
> by giving thanks, worshipping God.

Preparation

Arrange the room in circular seating. Reserve a space within the room for ritual prayer. Create an ambience for prayer with an artistic arrangement of the Easter candle, table, cloth, opened Bible, pitcher of water and basin, towel, and a living plant.

The day before the session, the persons proclaiming the word and those preparing refreshments are called to confirm their readiness. The materials needed are: Easter candle, table, cloth, Bible, basin and pitcher of water, towels, a living plant, song books, cassette player/tapes, matches, movable chalk board/chalk/eraser, catechist's notes, handouts and refreshments.

The Catechetical Session

Welcome

The participants and catechist greet one another by name and visit until it is time for the session. The catechist invites all to be seated.

Gathering Prayer

Catechist: Let us ask God to bless our gathering. (Pause)
(Gesture with open hands and arms outstretched.)
The Lord be with you.

All: And also with you.

Catechist: Let us pray. (Pause)
God of Community: Creator, Redeemer, Spirit, you are one in love.
Enable us to accept one another as we are, to bond through reconciliation and to serve those in need.
We ask this blessing in the name of Jesus, through the power of the Holy Spirit.

All: Amen.

Life Experience

Catechist: What goes on among people mainly determines what happens to them as individuals. What people know and believe, and how they handle their differences, begins in the family. You watched the film *Places in the Heart,* which depicts a portrait of a time and a place and a people, a family. It does this by entering the lives of specific families, families torn and rebirthed, and a family bonded in ways other than blood. (Open Discussion of the Film)

Discussion Questions: Class Preparation Handout
1. Who comprised the main characters of this human drama? How are we specifically introduced to these characters? Is there a basic human need revealed in these introductions?
2. What was the initial relationship of Edna, Mr. Will, Moses, Frank, and Possum?
3. What specific personal hardship did each central character experience in life? What experiences did they have in common?
4. How do these experiences shape each individual? How do they affect and alter the group?
5. Were there ever times in your life when you felt alienated or helpless? To whom did you turn to for support during these times of hardship? How were your nourished?
6. Can you recall times when you were there for others in need? In what ways did you reach out to nourish them? Did the experience transform your relationship? How?

Faith Reflection

Catechist: Table fellowship is characteristic of the ministry of Jesus. The Gospels tell of the significant meals Jesus ate with friends, sinners, the hungry crowds, marginal people, wedding guests, and with the disciples. Just like the bonding of the people in *Places in the Heart,* Jesus bonded with those whom he shared food, especially his disciples.

One meal that symbolized all the meals Jesus ever shared was the Last Supper of which he said, "I have greatly desired to eat this Passover with you before I suffer" (Lk. 22:15). This . . . meal was different than all the others Jesus shared. Why was it different?
(Open Discusion)

Possible Points of Discussion

1. Jesus made his life synonymous with the sharing of the bread and the cup:

   "Take this and eat, . . . this is my body." "All of you must drink from it, . . . for this is my blood . . . to be poured out . . ." (Mt. 26:26-28).

   "Do this in remembrance of me" (Lk. 22:19).

2. Jesus made Eucharist synonymous with service. In the Gospel of John (13:1-17), the story of Jesus washing the feet of his disciples replaces the narrative of institution of Eucharist.

   "What I just did was to give you an example: as I have done, so you must do" (v. 15).

Catechist: As ministers to the sick, we are among those who gather every Sunday to share the meal "in remembrance" of Jesus Christ. We are lucky to be able to come. There are some among us who cannot be present, namely, those who are sick. Therefore, we serve them and we care for them. We share the food from the table of celebration with them. We do what Jesus did. Taking the Word and the Bread to the sick is an act of service. Now, let us enjoy the refreshments prepared for us by (Names).
(Break)

Skills of Ministry

Catechist: The Liturgy of Holy Communion includes: the Lord's prayer, communion, silent prayer, and the prayer after communion. As presiders of prayer, let us first look to the skills of praying the Lord's Prayer with the sick. The Lord's Prayer is a prayer that is familiar to the sick person. It is a significant prayer. Say it slowly so they can follow along. If a person is very sick, the Lord's Prayer might be prayed as an echo prayer.

(Demonstrate) Repeat each phrase after me. Our Father (echo), who art in heaven (echo), etc. This skill takes concentration on your part. Practice with the person next to you. (Practice) By keeping the booklet, *Prayers of the Sick*,[46] with your rite booklet, you will have in print the common prayers the sick might ask you to pray with them.

In giving communion to the sick, take the lead of the sick person; watch for an indication to know if he or she prefers to receive in the hand or on the tongue. However, keep in mind that medication or anxiousness can dry the mouth. If this is the case, help the person with a drink of water first. Also, do not give communion to someone who is lying down. Put your hand under their back and raise them. If they are very ill, ask them how much of the host they can eat. Let them make the decision. If necessary, put water on a spoon and put a particle of the host in the water. Raise the person before giving them Eucharist. After the reception of Eucharist, maintain a few moments of silent prayer. Then, pray the prayer after communion and conclude with the blessing.

Please turn to page nine of *Communion of the Sick*. The rite (#74) tells us how those who are with the sick prepare for the liturgy of the sick; "prepare a table covered with . . . cloth upon which the blessed sacrament will be placed." Place "lighted candles" on the table and have a small "vessel of holy water." If those caring for the sick are unable to do this, the minister needs to see to these preparations. If in the hospital, use the bedside table. Bring a small cloth for the table. Place the pyx and a small candle on the cloth. The underlying message of the lighted candle is the remembrance of the Paschal Candle, the remembrance of the Risen Christ.

When you arrive to preside at the rite of communion of the sick you should be prepared. On entering the room introduce yourself and tell the sick person you are from the parish. If you know one another, greet the person and engage them in a few words. Keep in mind the scheduled amount of time. You set the boundaries; this is a skill. The person may want to hold you there. They desire your presence because they are lonely. You develop your own style of ministry according

---

46. Gabe Huck, ed., *Prayers of the Sick* (Chicago: Liturgy Training Publications, 1981), 1-48.

74 \ Eucharistic Ministry to the Sick

to your gifts and talents. The greeting and short chat establishes a pastoral presence. Then make a definite beginning of the rite.

Taking a current parish bulletin to the sick keeps them in touch with the happenings in the parish. If the person has not been on the parish sick list before, take her or him the parish gift of *Prayers of the Sick.*

Just Service

Catechist: In this session, we explored what it means to belong to a family. As unique individuals, the Lord calls us to unite as a Christian community. In nourishing us, Christ Jesus unites us to himself and one another. He calls us to the role of servant that we might nourish each other, most especially the poor and the sick. You have prepared to be a Eucharistic minister of the sick.

You have studied the rite, reflecting on its meaning in our lives of faith and achieving a familiarity with it to enable you to preside. Underlying your service to the sick is the fact that Jesus gave his life as nourishment *for all.* To do what Jesus did is to reach out to the sick in their specific need. It is to assure the sick of their rightful nourishment of the Word and the Bread from the table of the celebrating community of which they belong. We are responsible for their nourishment from the common table.

Preparation for Next Session

Catechist: Next week, we will share a potluck meal and spend time in prayer. (Name) has graciously volunteered to coordinate the food.

Ritual Prayer

(Catechist invites everyone to move to the prayer space. Participants are given copies of the psalm.)

Call to Prayer

Catechist: Where charity and love are found, there is God.

A Catechetical Process for Preparing Ministers to the Sick / 75

Let us remind ourselves of this in song.

Gathering Song

"Ubi Caritas"[47] (Taize)

Psalmody

    All: O God, your faithfulness endures forever.

Side One: Praise our God, all you nations. Acclaim the Most High, all you peoples.

Side Two: For great is your love for us; And your faithfulness endures forever.

Side One: Glory to you, Source of all Being, Eternal word and Holy Spirit.

Side Two: As it was in the beginning, is now and ever shall be. Amen. (Ps. 117)

    All: O God, your faithfulness endures forever.

Gospel Acclamation

(Sing along on the refrain: "People of God/Alleluia" (Celtic)[48]

Scriptural Reading

(Catechist lights the Easter candle.)

    Lector: A reading from the Gospels of Matthew, Luke, and John.

    All: Praise to you Lord, Jesus Christ.

    Lector: Do this as a remembrance of me (Lk. 22:19). (Gesture for all to repeat response.)
    During the meal Jesus took bread, blessed it, broke it, and gave it to his disciples.

    Jesus: "Take this and eat it; . . . this is my body."

    Lector: Then he took a cup, gave thanks, and gave it to them.

---

47. Robert J. Batastini, General Editor, *Worship* (Chicago: GIA Publications, Inc., 1986), 604.
48. David Haas, *Who Calls You by Name* Vol. II, produced and directed by David Haas and Kate Cuddy (Chicago: GIA Publications, Inc., 1985), audiocassette.

Jesus: "All of you must drink from it, for this is my blood, . . . to be poured out in behalf of many for the forgiveness of sins (Mt. 26:26-28). (Pause)

Lector: Do this in remembrance of me. (Gesture all to respond.)

Lector: Jesus rose from the meal . . . picked up a towel and tied it around himself. Then he poured water into a basin and began to wash his disciples' feet and dry them with the towel. . . . (Pause)

Lector: Do this in remembrance of me. (Gesture all to respond.)

Jesus: "As I have done, so you must do" (Jn. 13:4-5, 15).

Lector: Do this in remembrance of me. (Gesture all to respond.)

Lector: The Gospel of the Lord.

All: Praise to You, Lord Jesus Christ.

Response to the Word

(Silent Reflection)

Petitions

Catechist: Through the inspiration of the Spirit, we present our needs to God, who would have us be God's people, one people. (Pause)
For leaders of nations, may they work in harmony for the good of the earth, we pray . . .

All: Lord, hear our prayer.

Catechist: For us, may we bring our gifts of service to the community, we pray . . .
For the sick, especially (Names of Parish Sick), we pray . . .
For what else shall we pray?

Catechist: As one people, we present our needs and praise.
We pray as Jesus taught us:

All: Our Father . . . (Echo Style)

Greeting of Peace

Catechist: Let us offer one another the peace of Christ.

Closing Prayer

Catechist: Wondrous God, You are the source of peace and joy.
We hope and pray as did Jesus, that we all may be one.
We ask this grace in the name of Jesus, through the power of the Holy Spirit.

All: Amen.

Blessing

(The catechist blesses the participants by signing the cross on the forehead with water while asking God's blessing upon the person.)

Catechist: May God bless you to remember, and the Spirit empower you to do what Jesus did.

Closing Song

"Whatsoever You Do"[49]

(The session ends. The catechist thanks all for coming and for their participation. The catechist bids them farewell.)

Session Four: The Community Reflects and Prays Together

Objectives

The liturgical catechesis of this session will provide opportunity for the participants to achieve these objectives in the experience of:

Community

by welcoming one another.
by sharing a meal.

Life

by enjoying food which gives life and nourishment.
by celebrating through meal the bonding of the human friendship that grew from attending the sessions.

---

49. John J. Limb, General Editor, *Music Issue* 1993 (Portland: Oregon Catholic Press, 1993), 542.

Faith

>by reflecting on the presence of Christ revealed to the disciples in the Emmaus story (Lk. 24:13-35).
>by pondering how the sick bring a new recognition of the presence of Christ to the ministers.
>by sharing reflections on the presence of Christ.

Justice

>by making a personal decision to serve as minister of Eucharist to the sick.

Ritual Prayer

>by praying together as community.
>by experiencing the supportive bond of communal prayer.
>by giving praise to God.

Preparation

Prepare a buffet table and a banquet table. Reserve a space within the room for ritual prayer. Create an ambience for prayer with an artistic arrangement of the Easter candle, table, cloth, open Bible, a living plant and a pitcher of water within a basin draped with a towel.

The day before the session, the persons proclaiming the word, the cantor, and those in charge of the buffet are called to confirm their readiness. The materials needed are: Easter candle, table, cloth, Bible, basin, pitcher of water, towel, matches, living plant, song books, casette player/tapes, catechist's notes, handouts, a sign up sheet for a designated Sunday Mass for commissioning, and the food and drink for the meal.

The Catechetical Session

Gathering

The participants and catechist greet one another by name, and visit until all have arrived and the buffet is ready. The catechist invites all to stand around the buffet table for the blessing of the meal.

Meal Blessing: "Bread of Life"[50]

Catechist: Jesus is the Bread of Life.
For this Gift
Let us give praise and thanks. (Adapted)

Sung Response: "Bread of Life"[51]

All: I am the Bread of Life,
bread broken that you may live.

Scriptural Reading: Jn. 6:27-35

Reader: Do not work for food that goes bad,
work for food that endures for eternal life.

All: Sung Response

Reader: Then they said to him,
"What must we do . . . to carry out God's work?"
Jesus gave them this answer,
"This is carrying out God's work:
you must believe in the one God has sent."

All: Sung Response

Reader: The true bread . . .
the bread of God
is the bread which comes down from heaven
and gives life to the world.

All: Sung Response

Reader: ". . . Give us that bread always." . . .

---

50. John P. Mossi and Suzanne Toolan, *Canticles and Gathering Prayers* (Winona: Saint Mary's Press, 1989), 132-133.

51. Suzanne Toolan, *Canticles* (Winona: Saint Mary's Press, 1989), audiocassette.

All: Sung Response

Reader: "I am the bread of life.
No one who comes to me will ever hunger;
no one who believes in me will ever thirst."

All: Sung Response

Catechist: Jesus, we now break bread
and share this meal.
May we be nourished with your life
and filled with the freedom of your Spirit.
In imitation of your mission and the Gospel
may we nourish one another, especially the
sick. (Adapted)

All: Sung Response

Meal

Catechist: Enjoy our feasting of food and friendship.

Reflection

(After The Meal)

Catechist: As minister, you enable the sick to encounter the presence of God through the Word, through the Bread of Eucharist, and through your person. When you help relate the story of the sick to the story of Jesus, you help them see God's presence in a different or new way in their lives. While the sick are finding God in this new way, are you relating your story to the story of the sick, to the story of Jesus? Are you finding God present in new ways? This is a disciple's challenge also. Christ's disciples did not recognize him on the road to Emmaus. He was always present but they had to discern the new mode of his presence in their lives. Here is a copy of Luke's Emmaus Story and some reflection questions? Be alone with the Word. You might choose a quiet spot in here, on the patio, or somewhere else in or around the church. Please return in fifteen minutes.

Reflection Questions

1. What factors kept the disciples from recognizing the presence of Jesus?
2. What happened on the journey that enabled the beginnings of awareness?
3. Ponder the moment of realization of Jesus' presence. Why did it occur? What was the effect on the disciples?
4. Some relationships or acquaintances seemingly do not point to the presence of God. Why not?
5. How will the sick bring a new recognition of the presence of Christ to us? What will be its effect?
   (Reflection)

Catechist: Those of you who feel comfortable about sharing are invited to do so in your small group.
(Small Group Sharing)

Ritual Prayer

(Catechist invites everyone to move to the prayer space.)

Call to Prayer

Catechist: God's presence is our source of life.
In song, let us praise God
who creates, sustains, and redeems us.

Gathering Song

"Song of God Among Us"[52]
(Call/Response Style: Cantor sings phrase one, all sing phrase two.)

Scriptural Reading

(Catechist lights the Easter candle and gestures all to be seated. Soft music will be played throughout the readings, reflection pauses, and slides of ministers in the parish visiting the sick.)
(Slides)

---

52. Gather, 154.

Reader One: Moved with compassion at the leper's request,
Jesus stretched out his hand,
and touched him . . . . (Mk. 1:41).
(Reflection Pause; Slides)

Reader Two: . . . love the Lord your God
. . . and your neighbor as yourself (Lk. 10:27). (Reflection Pause; Slides)

Reader One: The Spirit of the Lord . . .
has anointed me
to bring glad tidings to the poor (Lk. 4:18).
(Reflection Pause; Slides)

Reader Two: Jesus said, . . . I have given you an example:
as I have done, so you must do (Jn. 13:15).
(Reflection Pause; Slides)

Reader One: I was ill and you comforted me (Mt. 26:36).
(Reflection Pause; Slides; Pause)

Reader Two: The Gospel of the Lord.

All: Praise to You, Lord Jesus Christ.

Response to the Word

(Cantor sings the verses; all join in refrain.)
"We Have Seen and We Have Heard"[53]

Petitions

Catechist: Confirming our belief that God is ever present and ever solicitous for us, we present our needs to God. (Pause)
For openness to the presence of Christ in people and situations of our lives, we pray . . .

All: Lord, hear our prayer.

Catechist: For the sick, especially for (Names of Parish Sick), we pray . . .
For what else shall we pray?

---

53. David Haas, *Who Calls You by Name* Vol. II (Chicago: GIA Publications, Inc., 1991), 24-25.

Catechist: In gesture and in words Jesus taught us, we present our praise and needs:

All: Our Father[54]

Closing Prayer

Catechist: Companion God,
in you we live and move
and have our being.
Open our hearts to find you within us:
help us to be alive to what is hidden,
strong in what is fragile
and loving in what is resistant to you.
Enable us to know your presence in others,
especially in the sick.
We pray in the name of Jesus,
through the power of the Holy Spirit.

All: Amen.

Closing Song

"City of God"[55]

Catechist: Before leaving, please sign up for commissioning at one of the weekend Masses. Ideally, the rite of commissioning should occur at each Mass this Sunday so the entire community can participate in the celebration. For your information, there will be a bulletin announcement of your commissioning with a list of your names and a short explanation of your ministry. You can be prepared when parishioners bring your new ministry up in conversation. (Name) will be in contact with you for scheduling for ministry to the sick. I will be in contact with you about ongoing reflection sessions.

(The session ends. The catechist thanks all for coming and for their participation. The catechist bids them farewell.)

---

54. J. Michael Sparough, S.J., *The Body at Prayer II*, produced and directed by Michael Sparough and Bobby Fisher (Cincinnati: St. Anthony Messenger, 1987), audiocassette.

55. Gather, 294.

Conclusion

This resource has set forth a catechesis for Eucharistic ministers for pastoral care of the sick, with some reflections for those who visit persons with HIV and AIDS. Let us summarize several conclusions which are based on the historical research, the theological reflection on the rite, the structural study of the rite, and the catechetical method.

The History of the Rite

Drawn from the historical research of the rite, the first conclusion is that the practice of lay ministers of Eucharist is rooted in the early church tradition. The most noted verification of this assertion is Justin Martyr's *First Apology:* "deacons distribute the bread and wine; they also carry them to those who are absent."

The second historical conclusion is that this practice of the lay assembly taking communion home for the sick and the participation of the laity in Eucharist are parallel trends. History notes that when the early church tradition of the assembly participating in Eucharist waned, the custom of taking communion to the sick from the worshipping assembly waned. Conversely, the efforts of Vatican II led to the restoration of the participation of the assembly in eucharist. The restoration of lay Eucharistic ministry to the sick also occured at this time.

Theological Reflection on the Rite

Theological reflection revealed three insights. The first of these is that *The Rite of Communion of the Sick* is the continuation of the community's Eucharistic action. Thus, the sick are sacramentally united with Christ; they are reunited with the Christian assembly; and, they are united to the assembly's liturgical action.

Two other insights are closely related: the sick have the right to Eucharist and the parish is responsible for the care of its sick members. Because the sick "are deprived of their rightful and accustomed place in the Eucharistic community" (RCS 73), "ministry to the sick is the common responsibility of all Christians . . ." (PCS 43). According to Mitchell, the pastoral principle, "to make the Eucharist as widely available as possible to those who reasonably desire it," determines who should distribute communion.[1] So, in the ministry of the sick, the legitimate need of those being served is the important issue. Those who are sick have the right to participate fully in the Eucharist through sacramental communion. Vatican II refocused the Eucharistic ministry according to this need and restored the church's early tradition of lay ministers of Eucharist to bring communion to the sick.

The Structural Study of the Rite

The structural study of the rite points to two conclusions. First, *Rite of Communion of the Sick* provides communion to the sick within the context of the liturgy of the Word. Because the rite is the continuation of the community's Eucharistic action, it is consciously modeled on the unitive liturgies of word and table. This structure points to the significance of the intimate connection between the Word and Eucharist in the liturgy. Eucharistic nourishment is to be preceded by nourishment from the scriptures. Second, because the *Rite of Communion of the Sick* is a liturgy, it is celebrated with a community. Liturgy is the action of the assembly. For this reason, the liturgy of the sick is celebrated ordinarily with a community of family and friends.

The Catechetical Method

In designing the catechetical sessions, two principles emerged. The first is that the *Rite of Communion of the Sick* shapes the preparation of the ministers. The study of the ritual components of the rite forms the basis for catechesis. The actions of gathering, listening to the Word, sharing the Bread, and being blessed – understood in their human, biblical, and ecclesial settings – are necessary to understand the whole liturgy of the sick. The study of prayer texts gives ministers an opportunity to clarify their theological understanding particular to this rite.

---

1. Mitchell, 282.

Pondering the scriptures of the rite enables the ministers to proclaim the Word to the sick and reflect that Word to their present human experience.

The second principle is that reflection on human sickness enables the ministers to be attentive to the needs of the sick. The liturgy of the sick celebrates the experience of human sickness. Preparing to preside at this liturgy necessitates a sensitivity to human sickness. Reflection on sickness gives the ministers understanding of the sick, and also suggests ways of relating to them and praying with them.

The parish community needs to be aware of its ministry to the sick, including those who suffer the double bind of being sick and also being rejected, as is the case for many people with HIV and AIDS. A brief list of resources for ministry to people with HIV and AIDS is included (see Appendix G).

In using the rite for sending Eucharistic ministers from the assembly to take communion to the sick, the community becomes aware of its ministry and of the unity created by this action. The prayer texts of the rite disclose this understanding:

> The celebrant addresses the congregation in these or similar words: The special ministers of communion will take Eucharist to those who are confined to their homes. [If possible, name the sick.]
>
> The celebrant addresses the ministers of communion: As you go, take with you not only the sacrament we have celebrated, but also the Word of God which we have heard, as well as the affection of this parish community, and ask for the prayers of those whom you visit in return.[2]

In this liturgical action of sending, and in the liturgy of communion to the sick, everyone is called to deepen his or her faith: the sick, the Eucharistic ministers, and the assembled community.

---

2. Gusmer, 197.

APPENDIX A

Analysis of Prayer Texts and Dialogical Exchanges

Rite of Communion of the Sick in Ordinary Circumstances

Text	Prayer	Address	Name of God	Description
81A	The peace	Community	the Lord	(God of) peace
	And also	Community	—	—
82A	Let this	Community	—	—
83A	My brothers	Community	—	—
	Lord Jesus	Lord Jesus	—	—
	May almighty	Community	God	almighty
	Amen	Community	—	—
86	Gen. Inter.	Lord	Lord	—
87A	Now let us	Community	—	—
	Our Father	Our Father	Our Father	Our Father who is in heaven
88B	This is	Community	—	—
	Lord	Lord	—	—
	Body (Blood)	Community	—	—
	Amen	Community	—	—
90B	All-powerful	God	God	all-powerful
	Amen	God	—	—
91B	May God	Community	God	almighty
			Father	merciful
			Son	
	Amen	Community	—	—

88 \ *Eucharistic Ministry to the Sick*

Text	Prayer	Deeds of God	Name of Jesus	Jesus/Church
81A	The peace And also	— —	— —	— —
82A	Let this	—	Christ	(Redeemer)
83A	My brothers Lord Jesus	— —	— Lord Jesus (3x) Lord (4x) Christ (2x)	— — — —
	May almighty Amen	— 	— —	— —
86	Gen. Inter.	—	—	—
87A	Now let us Our Father	 —	Christ the Lord —	— —
88B	This is Lord Body (Blood) Amen	 —	Lamb of God Lord Christ —	— — —
90B	All- powerful Amen	you nour- ish us through your holy gifts —	Jesus the Christ —	— —
91B	May God Amen	— 	Son 	—

Text	Prayer	Reference To Paschal Mystery	Spirit-Name/Work	
81A	The peace	—	—	—
	And also	—	—	—
82A	Let this	water calls to mind our baptism redeemed by death/resurrection	—	—
83A	My brothers	This celebration (Eucharist)	—	—
	Lord Jesus	Lord Jesus: healed the the sick forgave sinners gave yourself to heal us and bring us strength	—	—
	May almighty	—	—	—
	Amen	—	—	—
86	Gen. Inter.	—	—	—
87A	Now let us	Christ taught us to pray	—	—
	Our Father	your Kingdom come forgive us our trespasses	—	—
88B	This is	Lamb of God takes away the sins of the world	—	—
	Lord	your word heals	—	—
	Body (Blood)	—	—	—
	Amen	—	—	—
90B	All-powerful	—	your Spirit	—
	Amen	—	—	—
91B	May God	—	—	—
	Amen	—	—	—

Text	Prayer	Church	Petitions	Human
81A	The peace	you (sick/com.)	—	—
	And also	—	—	—
82A	Let this	us (the redeemed)	—	—
83A	My brothers	brothers/sisters	—	—
	Lord Jesus	us (sinners)	have mercy (6x)	—
	May almighty	us (sinners)	forgive us sins	—
	Amen	—	—	—
86	Gen. Inter.	—	hear our prayer	—
87A	Now let us	—	—	—
	Our Father	—	hallowed be your name	—
			your kingdom come	
			your will be done	
		us (needy)	give us daily bread	
		us (sinners)	forgive us trespasses	
		we (forgiven)	as we forgive	
		us (tempted)	lead us not into temptation	
			but deliver us from evil	
88B	This is	happy/we called	—	—
	Lord	—	say word/heal	I/un-worthy
	Body (Blood)	—	—	
	Amen	—	—	—
90B	All-powerful	—	pour our your Spirit – Keep us single-minded in your service	—
	Amen	—	—	—
91B	May God	—	God bless and protect us	—
	Amen	—	—	—

APPENDIX B

Lectionary Analysis

Rite of Communion of the Sick in Ordinary Circumstances

Lection	Form	Images of God	Reference to Sharing Nourishment of Unity
Jn 6:51	discourse: Jesus as bread	Jesus living bread from heaven	Anyone who eats this bread will live forever.
Jn 6:54-58	discourse: Jesus as bread	Jesus Father bread from heaven	One has life eternal . . . for my flesh is real food and my blood is real drink.
Jn 14:6	farewell discourse of Jesus	Jesus: the way the truth the life	Jesus is the source of life and truth.
Jn 15:5	monologue metaphor	Jesus the vine	Living in Jesus is nourishment from the Vine.
1 Jn 4:16	apostolic teaching	God love	Abiding in love is abiding in God who renews and refreshes.

Eucharistic Ministry to the Sick

Lection	Relationship to Person/Community	Theme of Reading
Jn 6:51	Jesus gives bread . . . my flesh for life	Jesus is the Bread of Life.
Jn 6:54-58	The one who feeds on my flesh and drinks my blood: has life eternal; will be raised up on the last day; and, remains in Jesus and Jesus in that one.	Whoever eats this bread has eternal life.
Jn 14:6	Through faith, ones who know and see Jesus, come to know and see the Father.	All come to the Father through Jesus.
Jn 15:5	Those living in Jesus and he in them will have productive lives.	We remain in Jesus through love.
1 Jn 4:16	We have come to know and to believe in the love God has for us.	God is love.

APPENDIX C

Human Sickness and Its Meaning in the Mystery of Salvation

Suffering and illness have always been among the greatest problems that trouble the human spirit. Christians feel and experience pain as do all other people; yet their faith helps them to grasp the mystery of suffering and to bear their pain with courage. From Christ's words, Christians know that sickness has meaning and value for their own salvation and for the salvation of the world. They also know that Christ, who during his life often visited and healed the sick, loves them in their illness.

Although closely linked with the human condition, sickness cannot be regarded as a punishment inflicted on individuals for personal sins (Jn. 9:3). Christ himself, who is without sin, in fulfilling the words of Isaiah took on all the wounds of his passion and shared in all human pain (Isaiah 53:4-5). Christ is still pained and tormented in his members, made like him. Still, our afflictions seem but momentary and slight when compared to the greatness of the eternal glory for which they prepare us (2 Cor. 4:17).

Part of the plan laid out by God's providence is that we should fight strenuously against all sickness and carefully seek the blessings of good health, so that we may fulfill our role in human society and in the church. Yet, we should always be prepared to fill up what is lacking in Christ's sufferings for the salvation of the world as we look forward to creation's being set free in the glory of the children of God (Col. 1:24; Rom. 8:19-21).

Moreover, the role of the sick in the church is to be a reminder to others of the essential or higher things. By their witness, those who are sick show that our mortal life must be redeemed through the mystery of Christ's death and resurrection.

The sick person is not the only one who should fight against illness. Health care professionals and all who are devoted in any way to caring for the sick should consider it their duty to use all the means which in their judgment may help the sick, both physically and spiritually. In so doing, they are fulfilling the command of Christ to visit the sick, for Christ implied that those who visit the sick should be concerned for the whole person and offer both physical relief and spiritual comfort (Prae 1-4).

APPENDIX D

Outline of the Rite

Rite of Communion of the Sick in Ordinary Circumstances

Introductory Rites

Greeting

Sprinkling with Holy Water

Penitential Rite

Liturgy of the Word

Reading

Response

General Intercessions

Liturgy of Holy Communion

The Lord's Prayer

Communion

Silent Prayer

Prayer after Communion

Concluding Rite

Blessing

APPENDIX E

Visual Aid for Session Two

Presence of Christ

... Christ is always present in his Church ...

... in the person of his minister ...

... under the Eucharistic elements ...

... when the holy Scriptures are read ...

... when the Church prays and sings ...

(CSL, 7)

APPENDIX F

Discussion Questions

Places in the Heart

Life Experience (Handout sheet)
1. Who are the main characters of this human drama? How are we specifically introduced to these characters? Is there a basic human need revealed in these introductions?
2. What was the initial relationship of Edna, Mr. Will, Moses, Frank, and Possum?
3. What specific personal hardship did each central character experience in life? What experiences did they have in common?
4. How do these experiences shape each individual? How do they affect and alter the group?
5. Were there ever times in your life when you felt alienated or helpless? To whom did you turn for support during these times of hardship? How were you nourished?
6. Can you recall times when you were there for others in need? In what ways did you reach out to nourish them? Did the experience transform your relationship? How?

APPENDIX G

A Brief List of Resources for Those Who Visit Persons with HIV or AIDS

Church Documents

A Call To Compassion, California Catholic Conference, 1987.

The Many Faces of AIDS: A Gospel Response, United States Catholic Conference Administrative Board, 1987.

Books

AIDS, The Spiritual Dilemma by John E. Fortunato, San Francisco, California, Harper & Row, 1987.

AIDS, The Ultimate Challenge by Elisabeth Kubler-Ross, New York, New York, Macmillan, 1987.

An Epistle of Comfort by William Josef Dobbels, S.J., Kansas City, Missouri, Sheed & Ward, 1990.

Prayer Journey for Persons With AIDS by Robert Nugent, St. Anthony Messenger Press, Cincinnati, Ohio, 1989.

The Color of Light: Meditations for All of Us Living With AIDS by Perry Tilleras, Minneapolis, Minnesota, Harper/Hazelden, 1988.

The Screaming Room by Barbara Peabody, San Diego, California, Oak Tree Publications, 1986.

The Walking Wounded by Beverly Barbo, P.O. Box 364, Lindsborg, Kansas, Carlsons',1987.

Voices of Strength and Hope for a Friend With AIDS by Joseph Gallagher, Kansas City, Missouri, Sheed & Ward, 1987 (tape, English and Spanish editions, Kansas City, Missouri, Credence Cassettes).

Booklets

AIDS and You: Facing the Facts by Daniel Grippo, St. Meinrad, Indiana, Abbey Press, 1995 (for teens)

When Someone You Love Has AIDS by Daniel Grippo, St. Meinrad, Indiana, Abbey Press, 1991

Organizations and Hotlines

AIDS Pastoral Care Network, 2931 N. Commonwealth, Chicago, IL 60657.

National AIDS Information Line, 24 hours a day: (800) 342-AIDS; in Spanish, (800) 344-7432; deaf access, (800) 243-7889 (TTY).

Consult your local library for additional resources.

Selected Bibliography

Church Documents

Catholic Biblical Association of America. *The New American Bible*. New York: Collins Publishers, 1976.

Flannery, O.P., Austin, General Editor. *Vatican Council II: The Conciliar and Post Conciliar Documents*. Vatican Collection, Vol. 1. Northport: Costello Publishing Company, 1988.

_____. *Vatican Council II: More Post Conciliar Documents*. Vatican Collection, Vol. 2. Collegeville: The Liturgical Press, 1982.

International Commission on English in the Liturgy. *Book of Blessings*. Collegeville: The Liturgical Press, 1989.

International Commission on English in the Liturgy. *Commentary: Pastoral Care of the Sick*. Washington, D.C.: United States Catholic Conference, 1983.

International Commission on English in the Liturgy. *The Rites of the Catholic Church*. New York: The Pueblo Publishing Company, 1990.

National Conference of Catholic Bishops. *Catholic Household Blessings & Prayers*. Washington, D.C.: United States Catholic Conference, 1988.

National Conference of Catholic Bishops. *Communion of the Sick*. Collegeville: The Liturgical Press, 1991.

National Conference of Catholic Bishops. *Eucharistic Worship and Devotion Outside Mass: Study Text 11*. Washington, D.C.: United States Catholic Conference, 1987.

National Conference of Catholic Bishops. *Sharing the Light of Faith: National Catechetical Directory for Catholics of the United States*. Washington, D.C.: United States Catholic Conference, 1978.

National Conference of Catholic Bishops. *Pastoral Care of the Sick and Dying: Study Text 2*. Washington, D.C.: United States Catholic Conference, 1984.

Books

Ahlstrom, Michael, Peter Gilmour, and Robert Tuzik. A *Companion to Pastoral Care of the* Sick. Chicago: Liturgical Training Publication, 1990.

Batastini, Robert J., General Editor. Gather. Chicago: GIA Publications, Inc., 1988.

Belford, William J. *Special Ministers of the Eucharist.* Collegeville: Liturgical Press, 1990.

Bergant, C.S.A., Dianne and Robert J. Karris, O.F.M., eds. *The Collegeville Bible Commentary.* Collegeville: The Liturgical Press, 1989.

Borrelli, Susan. *With Care: Reflections of a Minister to the* Sick. Chicago: Liturgy Training Publication, 1980.

Brisbane Liturgical Commission. *One Bread One Cup: Ministers Handbook.* Brisbane: Leader Press, 1982.

Brown, S.S., Raymond E., Joseph Fitzmyer, S.J. and Roland E. Murphy, O.Carm., eds. The *New Jerome Biblical Commentary.* Englewood Cliffs: Prentice Hall, 1990.

Cabie, Robert. *The Eucharist.* Translated by Matthew J. O'Connell. The Church at Prayer, Vol. 2. Edited by A.G. Martimort. Collegeville: The Liturgical Press, 1986.

Champlin, Joseph M. *An Important Office of Immense Love: A Handbook for Eucharistic Ministers.* New York: Paulist Press, 1984.

Dallen, James. *Gathering for Eucharist: A Theology of Sunday Assembly.* Daytona Beach: Pastoral Arts Associate of North America, 1982.

Deiss, Lucien, C.S.Sp. *Springtime of the Liturgy.* Translated by Matthew J. O'Connell. Collegeville: The Liturgical Press, 1980.

Fehren, Henry. *Is There Anyone Sick Among You?* New York: Pueblo Publishing Company, 1984.

Fichter, S.J., Joseph H. *Healing Ministries: Conversations* on *the Spiritual Dimensions of Health Care.* New York: Paulist Press, 1986.

Gusmer, Charles W. And *You Visited Me: Sacramental Ministry to the Sick and Dying.* Studies in the Reformed Rites of the Catholic Church, Vol. 4. New York: Pueblo Publishing Company, 1989.

Guzie, S.J., Tad W. *Jesus and the Eucharist.* New York: Paulist Press, 1974.

Haas, David. *Who Calls You by* Name. Chicago: GIA Publications, Inc., 1988.

Haas, David. *Who Calls You by Name.* Vol. II. Chicago: GIA Publications, Inc., 1991.

Hayes, O.S.F., Helen and Cornelius J. van der Poel, C.S.Sp., eds. *Health Care Ministry: A Handbook for Chaplains.* New York: Paulist Press, 1990.

Huck, Gabe. *Liturgy with Grace and Style.* Chicago: Liturgy Training Publications, 1984.

Huck, Gabe, ed. *Prayers of the* Sick. Chicago: Liturgy Training Publications, 1981.

Irwin, Kevin W. *Liturgy, Prayer and Spirituality.* Ramsey: Paulist Press, 1984.

Jungmann, S.J., Joseph A. The *Mass of the Roman Rite: Its Origins and Development.* Vol. I, II. Translated by Francis A. Brunner, C.S.S.R. Westminster: Christian Classics, Inc., 1986.

Keifer, Ralph A. *To Give Thanks and Praise.* Washington, D.C.: The Pastoral Press, 1986.

Kofler, Marilyn and Kevin O'Connor. *Handbook for Ministers of* Care. Chicago: Liturgical Training Publication, 1987.

Kubler-Ross, M.D., Elisabeth. *On Death and Dying.* New York: Macmillan Publishing Co., Inc., 1969.

Kwatera, O.S.B., Michael. *The Ministry of Communion.* Collegeville: The Liturgical Press, 1983.

Limb, John J., General Editor. *Music Issue 1993.* Portland: Oregon Catholic Press, 1993.

Link, Mark, S.J. The *Catholic Vision.* Allen: Tabor Publishing, 1989.

Luebering, Carol. *Ministers of the Lord's Presence: Eucharistic Ministers' Edition.* Cincinnati: St. Anthony Messenger Press, 1990.

Luebering, Carol. *Ministers of the Lord's Presence: Lectors' Edition.* Cincinnati: St. Anthony Messenger Press, 1990.

Luebering, Carol. *Ministers of the Lord's Presence: Ushers' Edition.* Cincinnati: St. Anthony Messenger Press, 1990.

Mayer-Scheu, Josef. "Compassion and Death." In *Concilium.* Vol. 94, *The Experience of Dying,* eds. Norbert Greinacher and Alois Muller, 111-125. New York: Herder and Herder, 1974.

McBrien, Richard. *Ministry.* San Francisco: Harper and Row, 1987.

McGee, Nancy. *Health Care Ministers.* Minneapolis: Winston Press, Inc., 1983.

McGeehan, O.F.M., Jude. *Ministry to the Sick and Dying: The Pastoral Reflection Paper.* Chicago: Franciscan Herald Press, 1981.

Mitchell, O.S.B., Nathan. *Cult and Controversy: The Worship of the Eucharist Outside Mass.* New York: Pueblo Publishing Company, 1982.

Mongoven, O.P., Ph.D., Anne Marie and Maureen Gallagher, Ph.D. *Living Waters* Text 2. Allen, TX: Tabor Publishing, 1992.

Mossi, John P., and Suzanne Toolan. *Canticles and Gathering Prayers.* Winona: Saint Mary's Press, 1989.

Murphy-O'Connor, Jerome. "Eucharist and Community in First Corinthians." In *Living Bread, Saving Cup,* ed. Kevin Seasoltz, O.S.B., 1-30. Collegeville: The Liturgical Press, 1987.

Nouwen, Henri J.M. *Out of Solitude.* Notre Dame: Ave Maria Press, 1975.

Nouwen, Henri J.M. *The Way of the Heart.* New York: Ballantine Books, 1985.

Seasoltz, R. Kevin. "Justice and the Eucharist." In *Living Bread, Saving Cup,* ed. Kevin Seasoltz, O.S.B., 305-323. Collegeville: The Liturgical Press, 1987.

Seasoltz, R. Kevin. *The New Liturgy: A Documentation, 1903-1965.* New York: Herder and Herder, 1966.

Senior, C.P., Donald. "Jesus the Physician: What the Gospels Say About Healing." In *Catholic Update,* ed. Jack Wintz, O.F.M. Cincinnati: St. Anthony Messenger Press, 1990.

Shea, John. *Stories of God.* Chicago: The Thomas More Press, 1978.

Sloyan, Gerard S. "Overview of the Lectionary for Mass: Introduction." In *The Liturgy Documents: A Parish Resource,* ed. Elizabeth Hoffman, 118-123. Chicago: Liturgy Training Publications, 1991.

Articles

Clarke, William. "Comfort for the Afflicted." *The Way* 16 (July 1976): 199-207.

Davis, Robert C. "Prayer and Liturgy in the Sickroom." *Liturgy* 2, no. 2 (1982): 59-63.

De Couesnongle, O.P., Vincent. "Living and Preaching the Gospel of Mercy." *Doctrine and Life* 42, no. 7 (1992): 417421.

Duggan, Robert D. "Celebrating with the Sick." *Liturgy* 25, no. 2 (1980): 11-14.

Duggan, Robert D. "Sunday Eucharist: Theological Reflections." *Chicago Studies* 29, no. 3 (1990): 209-223.

Fellows, Bill. "Toward a Sacramentality of Sickness." *Modern Liturgy* 19, no. 8 (1992): 16-17.

Glenn, M. Jennifer. "Sickness and Symbol: The Promise of the Future." *Worship* 54 (September 1980): 397-411.

Jorgensen, Susan S. "Pastoral Care: Heart of All Ministry." *Modern Liturgy* 19, no. 6 (1992): 10-13.

Luebering, Carol. "Ministries to the Sick and Well." *Liturgy* 2, no. 2 (1982): 55-57.

Normile, Patricia. "Visiting the Sick: A Guide for Parish Ministers." *Church* 18, no. 2 (1992): 27-36.

Power, David N. "All Things Made New." *Liturgy* 2, no. 2 (1982): 7-11.

Ramshaw, Elaine J. "Seeing Wholeness in Brokenness." *Liturgy* 9, no. 4 (1991): 9-17.

Rys, John H. W. "Ministers of Healing and Pastoral Care." *Liturgy* 2, no. 2 (1982): 75-77.

Williams, Donna Reilly. "Making Volunteer Ministry Work." *Modern Liturgy* 19, no. 6 (1992): 14-16.

Sound Recordings

Haas, David. *Who Calls You by Name*. Produced and directed by David Haas and Barbara Conley. Chicago: GIA Publication, 1988. Audiocassette.

Haas, David. *Who Calls You by* Name. Vol. II. Produced and directed Sy David Haas and Kate Cuddy. Chicago: GIA Publication, 1991. Audiocassette.

Haugen, Marty. *Mass of* Creation. Chicago: GIA Publication, 1985- Audiocassette.

Keillor, Garrison. *News from Lake Wobegon: Spring*. Produced and directed by Lynne Cruise, Margaret Moos and Tom Mudge. Lake Wobegon: Minnesota Public Radio, 1983. Audiocassette.

Sparough, S.J., J. Michael. The *Body at Prayer II*. Produced and directed by Michael Sparough and Bobby Fisher. Cincinnati: St. Anthony Messenger, 1987. Audiocassette.

Talbot, John Michael. *Quiet Reflections*. Produced and directed by Billy Ray Hearn and Phil Perkins. Canoga Park: The Sparrow Corporation, 1987. Audiocassette.

Toolan, Suzanne. *Canticles*. Winona: Saint Mary's Press, 1989. Audiocassette.

Video Recordings

Benton, Robert. *Places in the* Heart. Produced and directed by Arlene Donovan and Robert Benton. CBS/Fox Video, 1984. Motion picture.